The Magic Moment

To Mart

Yours Annabella

The Magic Moment

All I can give her is the moment

LOUIS SERRABELLA

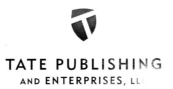

TATE PUBLISHING
AND ENTERPRISES, LLC

Published by Tate Publishing & Enterprises, LLC
127 E. Trade Center Terrace | Mustang, Oklahoma 73064 USA
1.888.361.9473 | www.tatepublishing.com

Tate Publishing is committed to excellence in the publishing industry. The company reflects the philosophy established by the founders, based on Psalm 68:11,
"The Lord gave the word and great was the company of those who published it."

Published in the United States of America

ISBN: 978-1-63185-370-8
Biography & Autobiography / General
14.06.06

To my wife Terry and my family—Jimmy, Jil, Jack

Contents

Prologue

Tomorrow is Valentine's Day, and I am standing in the greeting card aisle of our local supermarket attempting to choose a card that will adequately express the way I feel about my wife. She is standing passively beside me, but she is not at all aware of what I am doing. She wears the whisper of a smile on her face. It is the expression she wears most often now.

She appears to be content, but those eyes that once sparkled with intelligence and life are now blandly serene. I really doubt that she is very much aware of her condition or that anything at all is wrong, even though she has been told by her doctor that she has Alzheimer's. I believe she has either rejected the idea or completely forgotten it. Tomorrow I will give her the card along with a small box of candy. It is not the gift I would like to present her with. No, I would have preferred something more lasting and expensive.

Yes, I feel badly and guilty about it, as though I am somehow deceiving or cheating her. The truth is that I do not allow her to wear too much jewelry anymore because she has lost quite a few pieces including her wedding ring. I feel it would be foolish of me to continue buying more for her.

It will be necessary for me to read the card for her because her mind is no longer capable of comprehending what her eyes are seeing, and she cannot read. She will give me a big smile of pleasure, but she will not have the presence of mind to reward me with a hug or a kiss. If I am lucky, she may think to say thank you. It is all right if she does not. I understand. The smile on her face is reward enough for me. In a few short moments, she will have forgotten that I gave her anything at all. All I can give her now is the moment.

As I stood in the aisle reading through the cards, searching to find the perfect card for her, it occurred to me how vastly different the relationship between couples must be. Some of the cards were flowery and romantic, others were humorous, and some were quite sexy. I realized that the greeting card companies were cleverly offering a way that would enable each individual to express their feeling in a way that was most comfortable for them. No matter which category you chose, the message was very clear. Each card in its own way was saying "I love You." Most of what I have read and heard has been very helpful and useful, but while there are many similarities in all cases and certain methods of caring for a loved one that should be adhered to, we must, in the long run, be able to adjust according to our own personalities and relationships.

I am now a certified facilitator with the Alzheimer's Association and president of a large support group that meets once a week. We council, console, and offer encouragement to caregivers whose loved ones are in the various stages of Alzheimer's.

Come walk down the paths of my memories with me and I will tell you our own personal love story and the beauty and blessings of a closely knit family. As we stroll along, you will certainly enjoy the fragrance of the good times we had and perhaps grieve at the foul odor of the tragic disease that had so unexpectedly entered our lives. Perhaps those of you in my generation, and even those of you who came along a bit later, will find yourselves able to share a good chuckle with me at the humorous events. Then again, there may be a few paragraphs that might possibly cause a tear to fall. Perhaps you wonder what the *magic moment* is. I believe it will give you a better understanding if you simply read on and allow its meaning to unfold as I narrate my story.

How We Met

I was in a foul mood as I contemplated how unfair life could be. I had thought of little else for two years but how great it would be when I was discharged from the service and return home to my family. I was, of course, happy to be home again, but now I surprisingly found myself missing the life I had adjusted to in the navy. I missed the friends I had lived with in cramped quarters all those months, and the excitement of visiting a new port in a strange country. Now that I was once again a civilian, I found myself restless, bored, and lost. I knew what the trouble was, at least I thought I did. All my young life someone had taken care of me and told me what to do, first my family and then the navy. I desperately wanted to be my own man, to be independent and to be able to take care of myself. I felt helpless and frustrated. I had never given any thought as to how difficult getting started with my life would be in the postwar world. It was late afternoon, and I had sullenly retreated to my bedroom and flopped on my bed. I lay on my back with my left forearm covering my eyes while I mournfully considered what I could do about my seemingly impossible situation. My parents must have realized how lost I was. My father had served aboard a destroyer in WWI and had made several voyages across the Atlantic Ocean. He too must have experienced something similar to the despairing sense of uselessness that I was feeling now when he was discharged from the service. I cannot say, to his credit, that he ever pushed me, or made me feel anything but how glad he was to have me home safely again.

Mom too seemed to understand and being an Italian mother felt that the simple solution to all my problems could be easily solved if she prepared some of her wonderful Italian concoctions that were my favorite meals. She was certain that I had dreamed of these meals quite often while I was away, and she was right. "It's hard not to be happy with a full stomach," she would cheerfully state. Mom's given name was Amelia, but everyone called her Millie. Her parents, my grandparents, had migrated to the United States from Genoa, which is in the northern part of Italy. In the old days, the northern part of Italy had been invaded by the warlike Teutonic tribes of Germany. Probably for this reason, it was not unusual for northern Italians to have blue eyes and blonde hair. Mom had evidently inherited some of those blue eyes and blonde genes from her ancestors and was quite attractive. She came from a family of six siblings, four brothers and one sister. Because she was the oldest daughter, as was the custom in those days, it fell upon her to help her mother with her younger brothers and sister. She became a second mother to all of them, and even in the later years when they were all older, they would run to Millie if they became ill. She always seemed to know what to do and would nurse them back to health. Dad was good about it and even helped with the nursing. His father, my other grandfather, came from Spain, and he married a Belgium woman, my grandmother, who had both French and German blood coursing through her veins. I had fun telling people that I had enough different nationalities in my blood to start my own war. I sometimes wonder if the example they had set for me did not help influence me to accept my role as a caregiver later in life. It seems to have become a family trait. I tried not to show my despair and to pretend to be cheerful when I was around them, but I think they knew me too well to be fooled, and I realize now how it must have hurt them to see me this way.

I was disturbed from my reveries by the metallic ring of the telephone in the kitchen, and I heard my mom answer it. I didn't pay much attention to what she was saying as she chatted away with whoever it was that was calling. It was probably Grandma making her daily call to Mom, and those two would talk forever. I lay there half listening to the soothing murmur of my mother's voice as she spoke, and then after a few moments, she surprised me by calling out, "It's for you, Louis." Most of my friends just called me Lou, but my mom liked calling me Louis. "That's his name," she would insist indignantly if someone teased her about it.

"Who is it?" I asked.

"Come find out," she said with that little laugh that was always in her voice.

"Yeah, yeah, okay, I'll be right there," I answered.

I was feeling slightly annoyed at being disturbed from the preoccupation of feeling sorry for myself. It was my seventeen-year-old cousin who was all excited over having been asked to join a prestigious high school sorority. She told me the girls took turns having weekly meetings in their homes and that she was calling me up to invite me to stop by this Friday evening to meet some of her sorority sisters.

"It will be fun for you," she bubbled enthusiastically. "Lots of the boys will be stopping by after we are through with our meeting, and you would fit right in."

I hesitated for a moment. She was a good kid, and we were good friends. I really didn't want to hurt her feelings by refusing her offer, but I worried that the girls might be too young for a gnarled, world-wise, older veteran like me. After all, I had reached the very mature age of twenty.

I tried to gently voice my concerns.

"Gosh, I don't know, aren't the girls a little too young for me?"

"Hey, Lou, are you kidding? Most of the guys who will be there are veterans your age and older, you will probably remember some of them from high school."

What the heck, I thought. Her enthusiasm was infectious, and I was too darn broke to do much of anything else. I remembered one of my dad's favorite sayings: "As long as it isn't illegal, immoral, or too dangerous, always say yes. You'll have more fun that way." It had sounded like a pretty good piece of advice to me when I first heard him say it, and I still consider it to be a sage bit of wisdom to this day.

"Okay," I conceded. "It sounds like it might be fun at that, just tell me the time and the place."

She told me the meeting was at one of the homes of one of the girls who lived nearby and that it was close enough for me to walk to if I wanted to. She gave me the address along with the time the sorority meeting usually broke up and the guys were allowed to come over and come in.

I had been drafted into military service during WWII two months after my eighteenth birthday, and now, after having experienced military life, sailing the Pacific Ocean and making liberty in many ports, I considered myself an experienced man of the world.

In many ways, this was true. I had seen some of the seamier sides of life and had survived some difficult times. Life aboard ship was an environment that definitely required a man to be capable of taking care of himself or live a very miserable life. In retrospect, I realize now that although I had matured to quite some extent, there was still a good deal of that eighteen-year-old boy left in me. My despair was not unique, and I knew I was not alone in feeling lost. My boyhood buddies were trickling out of the service, and most of them had admitted to feeling the same way when we were able to get together for a few beers and complain about life. The job market was flooded with returning veterans now that the war was over. The defense plants on Long Island were no longer receiving those wartime contracts, and they were passing out pink slips to most of their old employees. Unemployment was high, and finding work was very hard, particularly for those of us too young to have any real marketable skills.

Most of us belonged to the "Fifty-two Twenty Club." For those of you too young to recall what this was, it was a government-subsidized program that gave the veterans $20 per week for fifty-two weeks or until they could find work. Twenty dollars week was almost enough to get by on in those days even if it was not exactly a fortune. We would take any odd jobs we could find and could just about get along, particularly if we still lived with Mom and Dad.

We were required to look for work and to submit a list of the places where we had applied when we picked up our checks every week. If you were fortunate enough to have a particular skill such as carpentry, auto mechanic, or electrician, you were not expected to apply for any other type of work. There was a story that circulated about one veteran who evidently was not exactly eager to find work. He insisted that he was an opera singer and would not accept any other type of work. I'll be darned if they didn't get him an audition with an opera company and found out he couldn't sing a note. I didn't know if this story was true or not, but it was always good for a laugh. At night, if we could find a few dollars between us, we would meet at the local tavern to have a few beers. We complained about our inability to find a decent job and were envious when we heard one of our acquaintances had the good fortune to actually have found employment.

We told sea stories about our adventures in the service and, of course, told vastly exaggerated tales of our many feminine conquests. We listened intently and nodded our heads in approval, but depending on who was telling the story, we suspected that many of the stories were no more than the wishful figments of the narrator's imagination. We were a ragged bunch. Most of us wore some part of our military apparel—blue jeans, army jackets, pea coats, and anything else that was serviceable. Many of us found that our old civilian clothing no longer fit us, and it was mostly for that reason that we continued to wear parts of our military uniforms. It was, in a way, part of our transition into civilian life. We were proud to be identified as a part of a huge fraternity of men who had served and defended their country during what we considered to be a just war. We were a proud and extremely patriotic generation. The transition from the service to civilian life was not easy. Many of us considered reenlistment, and a few of my friends actually did take this route. I too often thought of my hitch in the navy, and I knew it was not a bad life. Everything a young man could want was there—good food, medical care, and adventure. If you were ambitious and applied yourself, you could climb the ladder in the ranks and retire with a very nice pension. It was tempting, particularly since, as I mentioned, there seemed to be very little opportunity for employment presenting itself at home.

Of course the intelligent thing to do was to further your education by going back to school by taking advantage of the GI Bill of Rights. The GI bill was another government-sponsored program designed to give financial aid for education to the returning veterans. The longer the length of time you had served, the more points you gained toward the government paying for your education. Two years of service had not given me enough credits to complete a college education, so I decided to try photography school. I built a darkroom in my father's basement and became a pretty fair photographer. It was there that I developed the pictures I had taken of people's children, special parties, and anyone that would stand in front of my camera and allow me to earn a few dollars. It was a meager existence, but it did help to supplement my income and allow me to buy an occasional beer with the guys or see a movie. My parents asked me for nothing, and I felt terribly guilty that I was dependent on them to feed me and put a roof over my head. Is it any wonder that I was feeling deflated and depressed? I had reverted from manhood to being a little kid again. Now I found myself standing at the front door of some high school kid's home wondering what I was doing there. I rang the doorbell, and the door swung open almost immediately. A pretty teenage girl stood before me. She was dressed in the teenage style of the day—a plaid skirt, her father's long-sleeved white shirt with the sleeves rolled up, folded up socks, and what we called penny loafers on her feet. She was a true bobbysoxer. She looked me over, smiled, and said "Hi!" I returned her "Hi!" with a smile of my own and entered. I walked into a clean, well-kept, and comfortable-looking Victorian-style living room and was surprised at the amount of people there. I looked around and spotted several guys I recognized from high school, which immediately made me feel more at ease. I was about to walk over and say hello to them when my cousin caught sight of me and came rushing over.

"You made it," she gushed.

She then proceeded to take me by the hand and happily introduced me to several pretty girls. There was one in particular that caught my eye.

"Terry, I want you to meet my favorite cousin in the world. Lou, meet Terry."

I gazed down at a dark-haired, curly-headed teenager with a pair of big blue eyes that were gleaming with life. Whew! *I wish this one was a little older*, I thought.

I smiled politely at her, and in my very suave Brooklyn accent, I wowed her as I said, "Hi! Ya! How ya doing?"

I was really a smooth talker in those days.

She answered with a smile and a hi of her own. *Pretty little girl*, I thought, *going to be a heartbreaker in a couple of years*. That was that, and I guess it was not exactly love at first sight. My cousin and I moved along for more introductions. To my surprise, I found myself enjoying the evening, and after a few more meetings, I became a regular part of the crowd. We would go to various places like the beach or the local ice cream parlor to laugh and kid around. Most of the girls were still in their teens and too young to drink alcohol. Beer, of course, was the beverage of choice for the returning veterans, but heck, I had to admit that ice cream sodas were good too. I guess it was inevitable that some of the guys and girls would begin to pair off. Terry and I would see each other at these outings and say hi!, but that was about as far as it went. I was a little surprised when I became aware that lately every time we said hello, I was looking at her a little longer. I realized that I was beginning to think of her less as a cute kid and more as an attractive young lady. It occurred to me that one of these days, in the not-too-distant future, she was going to be all grown up. I wondered if it might not be a good idea to try and get to know her a little better now before someone else moved in ahead of me. I decided that the next time we all went to the beach, I would try to sit next to her and see if I could strike up a conversation with her. I was more than a little curious to find out more about what she was really like.

I soon discovered she was fun to be with. She had a great sense of humor with an infectious laugh, and she was smart as whip. My sailor buddies would have denied they ever knew me if I had not allowed myself to notice how good she looked in a bathing suit. *Shame on me*, I chided myself, *remember she is still just a kid*. It was probably more apparent to our friends than it was to us that we were beginning to enjoy each other's company. We just naturally seemed to gravitate toward each other when we went out with the crowd and found ourselves sitting together chatting, kidding around, and laughing.

I began to find myself thinking about her when we were apart and eagerly looking forward to when we would meet again. I rationalized that she wasn't too far from being eighteen and that dating her might not be too far out of line. After all, some of the guys were already dating girls her age and younger, and what harm could it really do?

She was just a cute kid whose company I enjoyed, and I was determined that I would behave myself. After all she was still young and jail bait.

I realized that the difference in our ages was the only thing that had foolishly prevented me from my asking her out. I had finally admitted to myself that she was almost constantly on my mind and there was little else I could think about. *The heck with the difference in our ages,* I prodded myself, *take a chance, call her up and ask her out.* I agonized for a day or two, and then I picked up the phone and dialed her number.

"Hello!" a young voice answered.

"Terry?" I asked.

"Yes, it is. Who is this?"

"It's Lou, how ya doing?"

"I'm doing good. How are you?"

"I'm doing good too. Listen, there is a pretty good movie at the Bayside Theater, and I was wondering if you would like to go and see it with me this Saturday." *My god,* I suddenly thought, *suppose she already has another date.* I held my breath as I waited for her answer.

"You mean like a real date?" she asked.

The question set me back, and I wasn't sure what she meant.

"Well, yeah, I guess that's what it would be," I ventured.

"I'd love to go, what time do you want me to be ready?"

I filled her in on the details, and we chatted for a while before we hung up. *Oh boy! Now what have I done?* She did seem real happy that I had called though. That alone made me feel glad that I had taken the plunge. *Come to think about it, I hadn't thought about reenlisting in the navy for quite a while now. Mmm! I wonder what changed my mind?*

Well, no big deal, just a date with a cute high school girl. Stop acting like you were a high school kid yourself with a crush, I mentally kicked myself. *You would think you never took a girl out before. Snap out of it.*

I can remember walking nonchalantly into my bedroom and accidently glancing into my bedroom mirror as I passed by. I really wasn't too surprised to find myself grinning from ear to ear like a complete idiot.

My Father's 1938 Chevy

This was great. Oh boy, now I had done it. I had made a date with Terry for Saturday night, and now I had to figure out a way to get my hands on a car to take her out in. I did not have a car of my own yet and was pretty much dependent on a few of my friends to provide transportation for me when we went out for an evening. Money was tight, and they were more than happy to give a ride to anyone that was willing to chip in and help buy a few gallons of gas. A full tank was an unheard-of luxury in those days.

I had been tempted to buy a car with the "mustering out" money I had received when I was discharged from the navy, but this was all the money I had, and I knew what an expense a car could be. Mustering out pay was a type of severance pay intended to help veterans get started after they were released from the service. I did eventually buy a used 1940 green Ford sedan when I found steady work and needed a car to commute.

I loved that little car, and I can still remember the thrill and sense of freedom I felt at the thought of owning my first car. I guess there is something special about that first car that none of us ever seem to forget.

Hitching a ride with my friends had worked out fine for me. It was usually just to go out and watch a high school football game, maybe for a beer, or perhaps a dance at the local park where there was no charge.

Because of this, there was no reason to ask my father for the use of the family car. But the truth was that the main consideration was that my father's 1938 black Chevy sedan was his pride and joy.

Please don't misunderstand me. Dad was a good guy, and we got along fine, but his car was his baby. It was washed and vacuumed every Sunday morning, and he kept it looking like new at all times. He had survived the Great Depression, and his few possessions had not been easy to come by. He appreciated and took good care of everything he owned.

Dad had what was considered a good job in those days. He was a top salesman for an old Brooklyn beer company called Trommer's Beer, and he considered his car to be an important part of his job and livelihood. The car was the sole mode by which he was able to travel his daily route and make his sales to the various delis and supermarkets.

I was pretty sure he would not refuse me if I asked him to lend his car to me, but I had tried to refrain from doing so because I understood, and respected, how necessary he felt his car was to him. Asking Terry out on a date had changed my thinking, and as much as I disliked putting him on the spot by asking for the use of his car, I knew I had to approach him cautiously and see what his reaction would be. I expected he would ask me what I wanted it for, and hoped he would understand my feelings, and consider my taking a girl out on a date an important enough reason. That evening, after we had finished dinner, I decided it was as good a time as any to drop the bomb on him.

I took a deep breath and spoke up, "Hey, Dad, I have a favor to ask of you."

"Sure, kid, what's up?"

I hated being called kid in those days, but I didn't think then would be the time to protest.

"I wondered if you would mind lending me your car this Saturday night," I blurted out nervously.

Even though he must have been expecting this moment for some time, the pleasant expression he had been wearing when we first started to speak suddenly collapsed into the look of man who had just been asked to take a large dose of castor oil. I heard my mother let out a small gasp, and her eyes were the size of saucers when I turned to look at her.

He was silent for a moment, he cleared his throat, and in a heavy and very serious voice, he asked, as I had expected, "What do you need it for?"

I felt a bit foolish, but I mustered up a smile and shyly spoke up, "Well, I met this girl that I kind of like, and I asked her out to see a movie with me this Saturday."

He was getting his composure back, and with some effort, he managed to return my smile. I knew Dad was a bit of a romantic. His family all spoke French fluently, which they had learned from their Belgian mother. They were highly demonstrative and loving. Hugs and kisses were routine, and romance was in their souls. I had heard the word *amore* spoken often as a child. I have to admit that all this had crossed my mind before I found the courage to ask for the car. Yes, I had given it quite some thought and was hoping that, between his Latin heritage and the French love of romance, he would not stand in my way.

He hesitated for a moment, and I saw his Adam's apple bob up and down as he swallowed hard and looked at me. This was my moment of truth.

"I guess it would be okay," he said, and then in a slightly ominous voice, "I know you will be careful with it, right, kid?"

"Thanks, Dad," I said. I had guessed right, and I barely was able to contain letting out a loud sigh of relief.

It was a cool Saturday evening in the fall, and there was a touch of winter in the air. The skies were overcast and gray as I drove my father's shiny black Chevy to pick Terry up at her home.

She must have been standing at the door waiting for me when I rang the bell because the door opened immediately and she came dashing out in her teenage attire. She was cute as a button, and there was no attempt on her part to hide her pleasure. She was absolutely without guile. I loved it.

I drove carefully over to the local movie theater and carefully parked the car. I looked to see that I was the proper distance from the curb and that there was a good distance between the cars. I was determined that my father would have his pride and joy returned to him in the same mint condition I had received it. Things had worked out well for me, and I wisely knew I would want to borrow the car again. I did not want to do anything that would give my father the slightest cause to refuse me at some later date when I wanted it again.

We walked up to ticket booth, and I bought two tickets. We walked down the aisle and found seats. The lights went out in the theater, and the screen lit up. The music started, and the show came on. After a few moments of indecision, I reluctantly reached in my pocket, pulled out my glasses, and put them on. I was slightly embarrassed at this admission of imperfection. I had a cousin who used to kid me by calling me "cousin weak eyes" after an old Al Capp comic character. I dreaded that Terry might possibly view me in the same way. She had never seen me wear glasses before, and I could not help but dread what her reaction might be.

I need not have worried. I heard her release a small sigh as she reached into her small purse and then with a tiny little girl giggle put on her own glasses. It was an ice breaker. I think somehow we felt closer as we shared one of our darkest and deepest secrets, and we both had to stifle a laugh as we looked at each other. Just imagine, we had discovered we both wore glasses, and it didn't matter at all. Actually, we both thought it was funny.

It seemed perfectly natural for me to put my arm over her shoulder as we sat there. It was no big deal. She certainly was not the first girl I had put my arm around, but when she made the simple gesture of moving a bit closer to me, I was surprised and thrilled at the foolish sense of pleasure I felt.

After the show, we stopped off at the local ice cream parlor and were not surprised to find several of our crowd there. They called us over to sit with them and good-naturedly teased us about our first date together. Terry actually blushed when one of the girls laughingly asked her if she was going to let me kiss her good night.

Two years in the navy had given me quite an education, and enabled me to become a bit worldly, but for my young date, it was really still a blissful world of innocence. I knew she had dated before and naturally surmised she had been kissed before. Why then, I wondered, had she actually blushed with embarrassment at the thought of kissing me?

I had the sudden realization that she was becoming very special to me. I hopefully contemplated that perhaps her embarrassment was because I was becoming someone special to her too. It was a very pleasant thought, and I grew quiet for a moment as I let it sink in. We had all heard people say that their heart skipped a beat at a moment such as this. I knew it sounded trite, but there might be some truth to this statement because I was sure that was exactly what mine did as I imagined what that kiss would be like.

Terry's curfew was getting close, and it was time for us to leave. It had started to drizzle as we left the ice cream parlor and headed for Terry's home. I turned the windshield wipers on as the rivulets of water began to course their jagged trail down the windshield. Visibility was becoming very difficult as the rain began to come down in buckets, and I strained to see the road.

I had noticed a trench crossing the road on our way to the ice cream parlor where evidently some road repair work had been done during the day. I had slowed down for it when I crossed it earlier, but it had been smooth, and I hardly felt it when I crossed it. Remembering this, I saw no reason to slow down for it on the way back.

The rain must have washed away some of the fill because the car hit the ditch with a hard bounce. I winced as I heard the sound of metal on the pavement. One of my hubcaps had fallen off and was rolling noisily, and merrily, down the road. I barely caught a glimpse of it out of the corner of my eye as it disappeared into a heavily weeded lot.

I had to get Terry home, and it was too late, too rainy, and too dark to try searching for the hubcap in that vacant lot with any hope of success. I dropped Terry off at her home and started to agonize over what my father's reaction would be when I told him I had lost one of his hubcaps.

I made it to my bedroom without disturbing him, although I was sure he was awake listening to hear me come in. I was relieved when he did not call out to say hello. I did not want to face him that night.

I woke up early the next morning and quickly dressed. It was Sunday, the rain had stopped, and it looked like it was going to be a nice day. I quietly slipped out of the house and drove my father's car back to the still wet and deserted lot.

Lying in the weeds, a few feet in, I could see the glint of a hubcap shining in the early morning sun. I smiled with relief as I walked over to pick it up. It was for a Ford.

Disappointed, I tossed it aside as I spied another hubcap in the weeds. This one was for a Buick. It was like a bad dream as I picked up hubcap after hubcap, all for various types of cars, but none for a 1938 Chevy.

I gathered up several hubcaps and put them in the trunk of the car. I wanted to offer some proof to my father that I had not been careless, and that I was not the only one who had been fooled by the bump. I hoped this would pacify him to some degree.

My father was peering nervously out the front window as I pulled his car into our driveway. I felt my stomach churn as I saw the expression on his face. Oh boy! I had taken his car out that morning without his permission, and he was not making any effort to hide his annoyance.

I beckoned him to come outside, and as he approached, I could see his countenance change from one of anger to one of concern. I realized he was visualizing a large dent somewhere on his beautiful car, and it was going to cost him a small fortune to repair it.

I quickly opened the trunk of the car before he could say anything. He stared in amazement as his eyes fell on the large assortment of hubcaps I had gathered. I explained what had happened to him and how his was the only hubcap I could not find.

Dad was not a man without a sense of humor, and I guess he could well imagine the concern I was feeling. His lips started to twitch, and suddenly he burst into laughter. I could feel the apprehension drain from my body, it was going to be all right, and in a few moments, we were both bent over, howling with uncontrollable laughter.

Monday morning, while traveling on his route, he stopped at an auto junkyard. He traded the hubcaps I had found for one that would fit his car. Later on in the week, I asked him if I could borrow his car again this Saturday. He looked up at me and said, "Sure, kid, no problem."

Come on now. If there is an ounce of romance in your bones, I know what you are probably wondering, and the answer is yes. I did get that good night kiss. It was a soft sweet kiss, and it was the first of many more.

It was a milestone event in our lives because, I know now, it was the night I began to realize I was falling in love with Terry. It is a sweet memory, and I am sure memories such as this are etched into the minds of most of us. This is only one small memory out of many experiences Terry and I have shared throughout the years we have been together. Ah! How wonderful it was to be young.

I believe that memories such as these are the yardstick that measures who we are and who we have become. To have lost almost all these events is almost like not having existed at all. Surely it is one of the most tragic symptoms of this horrible disease called Alzheimer's.

I continue to try to remind her of our life together, and she seems to enjoy my little stories. Sometimes they even seem to stir up vague memories, but usually she recalls very little and often disputes that they really ever happened.

On the few occasions when she does remember an incident, she is amazed that I know about that part of her life. She cannot fathom that the husband in the stories is me. I deeply mourn the loss of the loving partner I would have enjoyed sharing these memories with.

In a way, it is a blessing that she is not capable of feeling badly about the things she no longer can remember. She is not aware of what she is missing and seems happy and content for the most part. It is we, her family and friends, who love her, who feel her pain for her. Our life together has been a good trip, with just the right amount of bumps in the road to make us appreciate the smooth spots. Except for Terry's illness, there is not much I would change.

Falling in love with Terry gave me the impetus to get on with my life. I doubled my efforts to find employment. I tried my hand at various jobs, none of which offered much of a future. Eventually I found work in a supermarket that, at least, was steady employment. I worked in the produce department selling vegetables. The pay was a whopping $38 per week, but it enabled me to bring vegetables and meats home to my parents. It eased my guilt about living off them. I felt better about myself by just knowing I was making some small contribution toward my room and board.

I ran a lathe to turn down and shape musical clarinets out of some wood imported from Africa. Unfortunately, the wood stained my hands a deep brown that would not wash off no matter how hard I scrubbed. I even worked in construction, laying down water and drainage pipes and installing water meters. It was hard manual labor, but it put me in great shape.

I finally found gainful employment at one of the many defense plants on Long Island as a mechanical inspector. I had scored well in the aptitude tests the navy had given me, and they had sent me to basic engineering school. The schooling I received there had given me enough knowledge to be hired at a livable wage. I was able to advance myself by taking college courses in math, and other subjects that related to my job, in the evenings. Later on in life, I went into my own business in machining and electronic precision sheet metal.

In those days, as a couple grew closer, they would commit to each other by deciding to "go steady" and date each other exclusively. We were young, and Terry and I were deeply in love. We had gone steady for almost two years while our love for each other grew. I guess it was inevitable that we would begin to discuss the possibility of marriage. I was now earning a fair wage. Terry had graduated from high school and had a good job at a local bank. Things were looking up, and there was nothing standing in our way except for me to find the courage to ask her father's permission.

Terry and I nervously approached him, but there was nothing to fear. He had been expecting this moment for quite some time and was more than pleased to give us his permission. There was a certain warm satisfaction in the respect that was given and received by our generation. I occasionally see remnants of it today, but I fear, and regret, that most of it seems to have been lost.

We were wed one month short of Terry's twentieth birthday, and I had just turned twenty-three. To love, to honor, and to cherish, for better or for worse, in sickness and in health, till death do us part. At the time we both took our vows, we sincerely meant every word.

Before Terry

I have heard it said that we start to relive our lives again as we get on in years. I suspect that there may be some truth to this because of late I find myself recalling many incidents in my life, incidents that seem similar to those I am experiencing now.

The memories of these events, whether they are good or bad, seem to allow me to draw certain analogies that assist me in many of the decisions I must make, and attitudes I must adopt in my role as caregiver. To some degree, they have the effect of easing my mind as I go through the everyday stressful routine of caring for my wife. Because of these recollections, it often seems as though, as the old adage goes, "I have been there and done that before."

I grew up in a fairly good section of Brooklyn called Bay Ridge near the end of the Great Depression era. We were a semi tough bunch of kids who made our own fun by playing games in the street such as stickball. Stickball was baseball played with a broomstick and a rubber ball.

Kick the can and stoop ball were also popular games and lots of fun for kids who did not have everything money could buy.

Fences meant nothing to us, and although the school yard was locked up after hours, climbing in over the fence presented no problem if the urge came over us to play handball, shoot a few baskets, or occasionally get up a game of softball. Street games such as this cost nothing to play and were our primary source of diversion.

Money was something we had vaguely heard of but rarely came in contact with. By today's standards, I believe we would have been considered poor, but we all had a roof over our heads, and there was always food on the table. If we were poor, we never knew it.

My home was fairly close to the school, and if one of the kids fell down and skinned his knee or cut a finger, it fell on me to take him over to my house and put a Band-Aid on him. Most of the kids were a little squeamish about blood, and I suspect my little acts of first aid were one of the reasons I found a certain niche among my peers.

I smartened up and started to carry a few Band-Aids with me so that I would not have to run home every time someone shouted, "Call Louie, he'll fix it." As I look back, I sometimes wonder if my small acts of playing doctor were possibly something nurturing in my nature even at the tender age of ten or eleven years old.

We were really a pretty good group of kids who came from varied ethnic backgrounds. There were Italian, Irish, Polish, German, Jewish, and Swedish kids all attending the same school, and for the most part, we all got along fine. Of course, living in Brooklyn at our age there was, on occasion, the usual school yard fist fight after class, but it rarely had anything to do with prejudice. I do not recall ever hearing any one of my friends utter an ethnic insult or getting into any real trouble.

When I was about fifteen years old, my family moved out of Brooklyn to a town called Bayside on Long Island. Terry and I actually went to the same high school, but because of the difference in our ages, she was a freshman when I was a hotshot senior, and our paths never crossed.

Later on, when we were going together, her mom showed me some pictures of Terry when she was a freshman. Terry's mom was really a nice lady, but she was not noted for any great degree of tactfulness or sensitivity when she had something to say.

"I tell it like it is," she was fond of saying.

She had a great time teasing Terry about being all elbows and knobby knees in the pictures, much to Terry's distress. Terry was really a cute curly-haired little girl, but the pictures depicted her at that awkward age when most young girls hate their appearance the most. She was all teeth and bony angles. I made the brainless mistake of trying to please her mother by laughing along with her at Terry's discomfort. It was a bad move, and I learned something about feminine sensitivity that night. The lesson was driven home when the good night kiss I received that night was barely a brush of the lips that almost missed their mark completely. Oops!

I had entered the service soon after my eighteenth birthday and served a good part of my two years in the navy as a water tender in the fire room of an aircraft carrier called the USS *Boxer C.V.21*. I can still recall the evening I reported for active duty at Penn Station in New York City.

We were predominately young men in our late teens and early twenties. For many of us, it was our first time away from home and family. We milled about the huge lobby of Penn Station feeling lost and confused, our eyes darting nervously about as we searched for the sight of a familiar face from home.

Some of us tried to appear mature and unruffled by leaning against one of the large marble pillars that supported the high-domed ceiling and nonchalantly exhaled cigarette smoke through our nostrils. It is doubtful that we fooled anyone.

I had preferred to say my good-byes at home although my parents had begged to accompany me to the train station. I had felt it would be best not to prolong our farewell with the thirty-minute ride into the city trying to make small talk. I worried that watching them trying to be brave with tears in their eyes might be more than I would be able to bear.

As I stood alone in the crowded station, I glanced around and saw other men with their parents, wives, and girlfriends unashamedly saying their tearful good-byes. I could not help but wonder if I had made the right decision. I found myself missing my folks already, and I was beginning to regret not having agreed to let them come along to see me off. It would have been great for all of us to be together just a little while longer.

A very authoritative-looking uniformed chief petty officer spoke to us through a megaphone and ordered us to fall in while muster was called. We lined up in a very crooked unmilitary like line, smiling and feeling silly. I had a hard time believing any of this was real. I had the strange sensation that I was a little boy playing soldier in my backyard and that my mother would call me in for dinner at any moment.

After the roll was called, we were led down into the bowels of Penn Station where a long troop train awaited us. We had been told that our destination was a naval base called Sampson Naval Center on the Finger Lakes of New York.

It was September, and the city was beginning to turn dark by the time we boarded the train. I managed to find a window seat and threw my luggage on the rack above. I sat down feeling lonely and lost. Suddenly the train gave a lurch forward, and we began to move out of the station. I had the queasy, but oddly exhilarating, realization that we were very likely on our way to war.

As the train slowly began to pick up speed, I knew that with each turn of the wheels I was being taken farther and farther away from the people and things I had known and loved all my life. The similarities of the sensations and emotions I experienced then were close to those I feel now as my wife's caretaker. The only difference is that this time it is my wife who is going on a trip, not I, and I see my lifelong partner slowly drifting away from me on a train that no one has yet discovered a way to stop. I am told that there are ways to slow the train down so I can hopefully keep her with me for as long as possible. I voraciously read and research everything I can find on the subject of Alzheimer's. I want to learn what these ways are and work with the doctor to try them all. I watch carefully to see if any of the drugs prescribed work any better than the others.

I agonize, wondering if any improvement I think I see is real or if I am deluding myself. I want so desperately for something, anything, to help her. There are moments when it seems like she is improving, and I hold my breath. Can a miracle be occurring? The moment is always short-lived, and the train inexorably continues on its merciless journey.

I hopefully contemplate and pray that someone find a cure. Perhaps the answer is just around the next curve in the track. Alzheimer's disease is being studied, and new drugs are being tested all the time. Some of them quite promising.

Perhaps if the next curve in the track is not the answer, then the one after that just might produce the magic bullet we are looking for. The train still has some distance to go before it reaches its destination, I rationalize. Surely they will come up with something before it is too late. I could not live with myself or face my children if I knew I had left any stone unturned, and I grasp at every straw. I feel so helpless, and in spite of my every effort, there is still the gnawing sensation that I am missing something and I am letting her down.

Darkness had settled in, and lights were beginning to show in the windows of the apartment houses as we pulled out of Penn Station. Soon the big buildings were left behind as we traveled through the suburbs. The lights in the train dimmed for those of us who thought they might be able to seek the comfort of sleep.

A crap game started at one end of the car, and the noise they made cheering for their point made it almost impossible to do more than doze fitfully. Eventually the game broke up, and the steady cadence of the wheels clanking on the rails finally lulled me off into a restless sleep.

The sun was just below the horizon when I awoke, and signs of light were just beginning to try to show their welcoming beams above the now tree-lined skyline. The terrain had turned into rolling hills, and it appeared it was going to turn into a cold and overcast day. The view was mostly meadow land and wooded glens with an occasional house or barn dotting the landscape. The sight of those forlorn little buildings standing in the middle of nowhere seemed to emphasize the loneliness that many of us had coursing through us.

I was careful not to allow my inner feelings to show in any way. I instinctively knew that my transition from boy to man had to begin now. I kept my expression bland and even smiled occasionally to give everyone the impression that I was unconcerned. I have no doubt that many of the other men were trying to act out a similar charade.

It was early morning when we reached our destination and disembarked from the train. A heavy wind blew off the Finger Lakes, and the weather was turning cold as they marched us shivering to the induction center. We stood in a long line where we were each given an apple and a container of milk for breakfast.

They ordered us to strip, and we were walked through a long barrage of shower heads that were angled to strike us from every angle. They callously called it delousing.

We stood there naked and turning blue from the cold for what seemed like an eternity. The line we had been told to form began to move, and we were finally given clean towels to dry off with before receiving our uniforms and gear. The sailors passing out our uniforms would glance at us, and it was amazing how accurately they chose our sizes.

The two-story barracks they marched us to was cold and drafty. Later on when winter really set in, the temperature outside often dropped to below zero. The barracks never was able to warm up enough to keep us comfortable. Everyone soon developed a hacking cough, and the barracks soon earned the name of consumption ally.

I drew guard duty one night and was given a heavy baton to discourage any saboteurs or fifth columnists as we called them in those days. The navy had given us indoctrination talks, and I suspect that, half in jest, they convinced us that there were enemy agents out there whose primary purpose in life was to blow up one of our barracks.

I stationed myself at my post by the front door and sleepily leaned against the bulkhead. Time went by slowly, and it was all I could do to stay awake. Suddenly I was startled as the shadowy figure of a man loomed in the dimly lit doorway.

"Halt, who goes there?" I challenged as I had been instructed to do.

There was no answer. I loudly repeated my challenge, but there was still no answer as he kept advancing. I raised my baton to strike. There was no way someone was going to blow up my barracks while I was on guard duty. The supposed saboteur belatedly answered me in what sounded like a very unmilitary frightened voice when he saw me coming at him.

"It's only me, watsa matter with you, sailor?" he cried out as he stepped back to get away.

I recognized him then as the petty officer in charge of our company barracks. He was evidently returning from liberty and was more than a little bit under the weather. I wondered if I was in trouble, but he just staggered off to his quarters shaking his head. I wonder if he ever realized how close he came to getting knocked cold by a fledgling, frightened, and gullible young sailor. I never heard anything more about it, and I doubt, considering the shape he was in, that he even remembered it.

My watch was nearly over, and it was time to wake up my relief. Every man's bunk was numbered, and I had no difficulty in finding him in the dimly lit barracks. I found his bunk not too far from my own, and because it was a bit too early to wake him, I decided to let him sleep a while longer.

I could hear the men coughing and hacking in their bunks, miserable, and unable to sleep. My throat was tickling too, and I recalled that I had purchased some cough drops at navy stores earlier in the day. I walked over to my locker and popped one in my mouth to suck on while I undressed. I was pleased that the tickle in my throat eased almost immediately. I congratulated myself on my foresight and with youthful arrogance shook my head at the stupidity of the other men who had not thought to do the same.

I walked back to my relief's bunk and gently shook his feet to wake him. You were not allowed to touch any other part of a man when you had to wake him, just his feet. He woke up easily and slid out of his bunk with a small sigh.

"Consumption ally is living up to its name tonight," he commented, and I nodded my head in agreement. I did not tell him about my little adventure with the supposed fifth columnist.

He was one of the older men in the barracks, and we had nick named him Pops, after all he must have been twenty-nine or thirty years old. He opened his locker, and I noticed that he too had purchased a box of cough drops. He put one in his mouth, but instead of returning the box to his locker as I had done, he started to go from bunk to bunk passing out his remaining cough drops to the men who seemed to be suffering the most.

It was not exactly an earth-shattering gesture, but I was impressed with his generosity. I experienced a moment of guilt when I remembered my own reaction when I heard the men coughing. I had been smug and critical while he had reacted with compassion.

He finished dressing and with a little wave walked off to take his post at the front door. I lay there in my bunk contemplating the act of kindness I had just witnessed. Even though I was dead tired, I found myself turning, twisting, and unable to drift off to sleep.

It was no use. Try as I might, I could not rid myself of the guilt I was feeling. I finally and begrudgingly admitted to myself what I had to do if I was going to get any sleep that night. I rolled out of my bunk and went to my locker. I took out my box of cough drops. I hesitated for a moment, but I selfishly could not resist putting one under my pillow for later. Following the example of Pops, I dispersed my remaining cough drops to the suffering men.

"Thanks, mate," they would say, and after a while, as I lay in my bunk, it seemed to me that the coughing began to subside a little. I slept well.

I grew up a little that night and learned a valuable lesson about compassion. I also discovered how good a simple unselfish act can sometimes make you feel inside. Playing the role of caregiver can be quite demanding. It is similar to having a young child whose needs must be attended to at all times, a child whose behavior you know will never improve but can only worsen. I am human, and there are times, particularly when I am tired, that I succumb to moments of depression and crankiness. It is then that I am most prone to losing my patience. The guilt that I feel afterward makes me shrink with remorse. Fortunately she does not remember what I may have said for very long, and things go back to normal in a very short time.

I admit that there is a certain amount of self-delusion in my thinking, but to overcome my moodiness and regain my patience, I deliberately allow my mind to drift back to that night in the barracks. Of course the small deed I performed that night is nothing compared to the duties I must perform now in trying to care for my wife.

Perhaps my reasoning may seem odd to some, but is my thinking really something so bizarre? I find that recalling the events of that night takes my mind off my immediate problems and helps me to regain control of my emotions. I am able to calm myself and place each small chore I must do to help my wife in its proper perspective. I must remain positive and patient and think of each thing I do for her as no more than passing out another cough drop. If she were able to understand how much I am trying to help her, I am sure she too would say "Thanks, mate."

A World Of Beauty, A World Of Pain

The day finally came when boot camp was over and we were given ten days leave to be with our families before we were shipped out to wherever they had decided to send us. We were all excited at the prospect of going home but unfortunately my happiness was to be very short lived.

I did not realize it but "consumption alley" had taken its toll on me. I was not exactly feeling in the pink when I got home and was only able to eat a small token of the delicious meal my mother had prepared for me, much to her, and my disappointment. I was not feeling well at all, I was very tired and not at all my usual self. I chatted with my family for a while but I finally had to tell them that I was dead tired and needed a good night's sleep. We all surmised it was just the excitement of being home again. I said goodnight and disappointedly slowly walked into my old familiar bedroom.

The following morning when I awoke I found I could hardly move and was too weak to get up. I was sick as a dog. I called my father to my room and told him that I was ill.

"What do you want me to do?" he asked with concern.

"Call up St. Albans Naval Hospital and tell them I am on boot leave and have become ill. Ask them for instructions on what I should do."

I knew that St. Albans was not too far from our home and it seemed like my best bet. He was told to drive me to the hospital and was cautioned that I had better really be sick.

"He could be in real trouble if he is trying to goof off." They warned.

Dad drove me to the hospital, and I was diagnosed with pneumonia and immediately admitted for treatment.

I really had become quite sick and they did not have penicillin in those days. Sulfur drugs were the best they had to offer and although they worked fairly well on me, it took a while for me to recover.

After several weeks I eventually felt better and was gaining my strength back. I was able to get up and walk around to the hospital recreation room and visit with some of the men I had met.

One day we were told that they were going to have a dance in the gym the following Saturday afternoon. A few of us felt good enough to want to see some girls other than the nurses and thought we would give it a whirl. We walked into the gym that Saturday and looked around. Most of the girls seemed a bit older than we were and for some of the men that was a bit of a deterrent.

As I glanced around I was surprised to see a group of girls I knew from high school. They were all sisters in a sorority noted for the beauty of its members. I had always thought of them as girls that were way out of my reach and although I knew them all I had never tried to date any of them. It was the same sorority that my cousin had joined later on and that Terry too eventually belonged to when I first met her.

I pointed them out to my friends without saying I knew them. "Look at those good looking young chics over there."

"Should we ask them to dance?" I asked them.

"Do you think they would?" one of my buddy's asked.

"One way to find out." I said, and I bravely walked over to meet them. My buddies were stunned at my courage.

The girls recognized me and I was given a big greeting. They asked me what I was doing here and had I been wounded. It was tempting to make myself out as a wounded war hero but I told the truth. They did not look too disappointed that I had not seen action yet.

I guess it would have been nice for them if they could have told everyone they had danced with a wounded was hero they knew from high school.

I beckoned for my friends to come on over and I smilingly introduced everyone. The prettiest girl was a shapely blond with great big blue eyes and a smile that lit up the room. I chose her for myself. She was really very nice and not a bit stuck up over her beauty. It felt so good to dance with a pretty young girl again.

After the dance I was considered a hero by my buddy's and had all I could do to prevent them from carrying me out on their shoulders. I gained quite an undeserved reputation as a Don Juan that afternoon. Yeah, I loved it.

After a stint in rehab I was returned to active duty. I had scored well on my aptitude tests in boot camp and my next assignment was to attend basic engineering school at Great Lakes Naval Training Station and as I mentioned earlier, it was this training that enabled me to find decent employment later on. Both the time it took for me to recover from my illness, and the time it took for my schooling, delayed me from being shipped overseas for several months.

Upon the completion of my training I was sent by rail to San Francisco and placed aboard a slow moving troop transport ship bound for Honolulu. When we first moved out to sea from the port of San Francisco we cautiously moved out into the rough Pacific Ocean on high alert. We sailed with no running lights on in order to avoid presenting ourselves as an easy target for enemy submarines to torpedo.

San Francisco was blacked out so that our ships would not be silhouetted against lit city lights.

It was on the second or third day at sea, when we were about half way to Hawaii, that the public address system suddenly blared.

"Attention all hands, now hear this, now hear this."

The captains voice crackled with emotion as he announced that that Japan had surrendered unconditionally and the war was over. A loud roar resounded throughout the ship as we shook hands and slapped each other on the back.

We had overcome a formidable enemy and the world was at peace once again.

I doubt there was a man aboard the ship that did not jokingly brag that the Japanese had surrendered because they found out he was coming.

I was young and naïve and my idea of war was us shooting at the enemy. I knew they would shoot back but with youthful bravado and stupidity I considered myself invincible. It would be one of my mates who fell mortally wounded, and that bothered me, but certainly it would not be me.

I had mixed emotions, although I was elated that the war was over and felt a strong sense of relief, there was a part of me that was slightly disappointed at being too late to see any action. As I grew older and wiser later on, that gung ho attitude disappeared and I consider myself to have been very lucky.

We were billeted on Ford Island which was close to Honolulu for a short time. We made liberty in the city and saw sights such as Waikiki Beach. We played baseball at the base most afternoons and at the last minute would run for shelter as the afternoon rains approached us in a solid sheet of water.

A beautiful and majestic aircraft carrier pulled into port and we were thrilled to discover she was to be our ship. The carrier was a city within itself and had a population to match, It had a compliment of somewhere in the vicinity of about three thousand men. In the time I served aboard her I never did get to see the whole ship.

I was assigned to number one fire room which was a bit like being sent to hell. The temperature, because of the heat being emitted from the boilers, averaged about 120 degrees. We worked in six shifts which mercifully reduced the lengths of our watches to four hours. It was all a human being could handle efficiently.

It was rough duty down there because there was no air conditioning aboard navy ships in those days. Huge fans blew fresh air into the lower decks of the ship forcing it through large ducts. The fresh air did offer some relief but it too was warm by the time it reached us.

In time we all learned to acclimate ourselves to the heat and to drink the fire room coffee which was always tinted with the fowl taste of diesel oil fuel.

If a deckhand committed some infraction of the regulations it was considered very severe punishment for him to have to serve a watch with us. We laughed at their discomfort and the fact that we rarely saw the same deck hand again. Serving a watch with us was considered something that would deter anyone from making the same mistake twice. What they considered to be severe punishment was no more than what we did every day.

I am well aware that there were many men in the service who had to tolerate much worse situations than we did. That having been said, I doubt that any of us who served in that corner of Hades called the fire room who did not eventually become capable of adjusting to almost any adverse situation that life might send our way.

My ship mates were from every state in the union and from all walks of life. There were the clean cut somewhat innocent all American boys from good homes. There were the tough street wise kids from some of the worst neighborhoods in the country. Any sign of weakness among these men could make your life very miserable and you quickly learned to take care of yourself or else.

You put on a brave front and if you harbored any fears at all it was wise to keep them well hidden and never, never, never, back down.

The fire room was located deep in the bowels of the ship and well below the water line. It occurred to me that had we seen action, and taken a torpedo hit anywhere near the fire room, the chances of our getting above decks in order to survive were not very good.

It was then that I began to reconsider my former gung ho attitude. My earlier admission that perhaps my not seeing any action was an adventure I could gladly forego was re-enforced . As one of the men put it, "There are no roses on a sailors grave."

We sailed the Pacific and made ports of call at many exotic oriental cities and beautiful tropical islands. It was a million dollar adventure tour and we were privileged to visit such cities in China as Shanghai, Tsingtao, and Hong Kong. We strolled or rode in rickshaws along the crowded streets and were fascinated by some of the sights we saw.

When we glanced into an ally we could often see homeless people lying hopelessly among their few scant possessions. Many of them were obviously sick and starving, they were torn between desperately trying to survive and praying for a quick death to end their misery.

Disease was rampant and it was not an uncommon sight to see someone lying in the street dead or dying as their countrymen, simply stepped over or around them. They were viewed with distain by their own people who often wore surgical masks in order to prevent themselves from being exposed to any of the possibly contagious diseases.

Prostitution was everywhere and whores with young children would try to sell you a child for five dollars. They knew that no matter what the child's lot might be living with us, it had to be better than the life it had facing it in China. Some of the women were pregnant and could not ply their trade because no one wanted them in their condition. It was a cruel and meager existence these people endured.

In my youthful innocence it had never occurred to me that there were people in the world that were forced to live this way. We have all read about or seen pictures of this type of thing, but to actually witness the reality of something like this puts life in an entirely different perspective.

I have never been able to completely forget these terrible scenes, and when life occasionally seems to be intolerable for me, the vision of these poor unfortunate souls comes to my mind. My troubles become minimal by comparison and I can only bow my head and count my many blessings.

I had a very unpleasant lesson in life driven home to me when I discovered how difficult and cruel life can be. It was fortunate that I was able to offset the ugliness of these scenes with the natural beauty I was also exposed to.

Many of the tropical islands such as Guam and Saipan were so beautiful that they defied description There were white sandy beaches that seemed to travel endlessly in either direction, they lay there patiently waiting for the clear aquamarine water to lap gently upon their shores. Scores of palm trees, a few yards from the water's edge, stood silently swaying in the warm breeze and provided comforting shade and relief from the sun's rays.

Beyond the trees the jungle grew where the land had not yet been cleared. The warm sun beat mercilessly down on us and we dove into the water in an attempt to cool off. Water so clear that you could easily see bottom twenty feet down. We played water tag in water that was filled with hundreds of small multi colored, iridescent tropical fish, that darted swiftly between our legs as we swam. There were breathtaking sunrises and sunsets whose many hues and colors of orange, yellow and blue would defy any artists brush to ever truly capture them on canvas.

There were star filled nights when the moon was so enormous and bright that you could literally read a newspaper by its glow. These tropical islands could not help but enhance ones soul, and regardless of the misery we had seen in the Asian cities, we were reminded that there was also beauty everywhere in this world if only you were wise enough to look for it and astute enough to actually see it.

We sailed the Yellow Sea and although we could not see the mainland because we were too far off shore, we could usually detect the unpleasant and musty odor of the Chinese mainland. It was scent which I can only describe as a mixture of garlic and damp soil.

There were overcast days when the sea was as calm as a bath tub. The color of the sky and the sea would blend so perfectly that it became impossible to detect where one began and the other ended. The horizon became invisible and the water seemed to melt into the hazy sky. It was a scene that gave the eerie impression that the ship had left this world and was floating in space. It was quite a fantastic sight to behold.

If I let my imagination wander I could visualize an old sailing ship bursting out of the mist with cannons booming. It would be flying the Jolly Rodger and vicious looking Chinese pirates would be grimacing from the rigging with knives in their teeth.

We saw the devastation our bombs had wrought on cities such as Tokyo and Yokohama in Japan. We walked the streets and visited the bars that had risen out of the rubble. Japanese soldiers still in uniform glared at us as we walked by and we glared right back at them. Fortunately the glaring was as far as it ever went.

The day came when I had amassed enough points to be discharged. Once again I found myself billeted in Hawaii for a short time while I waited for a troop transport ship to take me stateside. I did not have to wait very long and I was soon back in San Francisco where I eventually boarded a troop train to take me cross country to my home and family.

The transport ship was an quite an interesting experience. Every evening after chow time the mess hall would be cleared and would suddenly turn into a gambling casino.

There was roulette, poker games, black jack and just about any game you wanted to gamble on. The dealers took ten percent of every pot and money flowed like water. I have no doubt that every crewman aboard that ship went home a rich man. It was interesting to note that the ships officers were never seen during these gambling hours. It did not take a genius to figure out they were getting their cut too.

The troop train that carried us across country to home consisted of boxcars which had been nicely renovated into very comfortable living quarters complete with double bunks and tables.

We opened the sliding doors sat with our legs dangling out so we could enjoy watching the countryside go flashing by. When the train chugged through the many small towns along the way we would hoot and whistle at any pretty girls we might see.

They were good natured and would laugh and wave back at us, after all, we were sailors and we had our reputation to uphold. They must have wondered where we had been, what we had seen and been through, and I am sure they were glad for us knowing we were finally returning safely to our homes.

I had written my folks that I was on my way home while I was in San Francisco but that I had no idea when I would show up. It was my intention to phone them when I arrived at Penn Station to let them know I was near.

When I reached Penn Station and disembarked from the troop train I was pleased to discover that there was a train leaving on the Long Island Railroad for Bayside in a few minutes. I decided to run for it which left me no time to make that phone call to my folks.

It had been a long time since I had been home and my excitement grew with every clanking sound the wheels made on the rails. The half hour ride seemed to take an eternity but the moment I had dreamed about and waited so long for finally arrived and I was pulling into Bayside Station.

I started to look for a pay phone so I could call my folks to come pick me up. I knew my father would have been there before I could hang up, but I was slightly overcome with nostalgia at the familiar sight of my home town.

As anxious as I was to see my folks again I decided to walk the short mile and one half home from the station. I wanted to enjoy seeing my old stomping grounds again and remembering the good times and places that I had once frequented.

I slung my duffle bag over my shoulder and eagerly started to walk the final leg of my long awaited journey home. It was a calm winter evening with hardly a breeze stirring.

I know it must sound unlikely, like something out of an old Bing Crosby Christmas movie, but a light snow really did begin to gently fall to the ground, some of it settling on the shoulders of my navy blue pea coat. Soon everything began to turn white and all was peaceful and serene.

I made my way along the familiar streets that I had traveled so many times before as a teenager. I met no one that I knew but strangers would smile broadly and nod at me as I walked down Bell Boulevard, which was Bayside's main street. The war was over and people were happy to see another service man returning home safely to his loved ones.

It had been about two years since I had been home. It didn't seem possible but there I was standing at the bottom of the steps that led to my front door. I climbed the steps and when I stood before the door I slowly reached out and pressed my finger against the doorbell.

My heart beat faster in anticipation as I heard footsteps approaching the door. I prepared myself for the big welcome I was sure I was about to receive.

My mother opened the door and looked at me with a pleasant smile.

"Yes." she said.

My God! I thought, have I changed that much that she doesn't recognize me? This was definitely not the homecoming reception that I had visualized and I was badly disappointed.

"Mom, it's me." I blurted out.

Her face contorted into one of amazement.

"Jim, Jim," she screamed for my father and suddenly threw herself into my arms.

"Oh my God! It's Louis and he's home." she shouted for him to hear.

I hugged her back as she cried with joy and showered my face with kisses.

I smilingly reached behind her so I could shake hands with my father. He had come running when she had called out and was enthusiastically trying pump my arm off as we shook hands. We were both beaming from ear to ear and I was not surprised to notice that there was a tear in the corner of his eye.

This was more like the welcome I had expected. The wonderful emotions I experienced that snowy winter evening are beyond my ability to express. All I could think of was I'm home, I'm home with my family, I'm home again at last.

The Accident

I was enjoying myself one lazy summer afternoon watching Jimmy Connors play in an exciting tennis match on TV when I heard the click of a key being inserted in the front door. It was followed immediately by the sound of the front door opening and closing. I knew it was Terry returning from her usual Saturday afternoon shopping spree. I turned my head expectantly toward the hallway as I waited for her to shout her usual greeting.

"Halloo, anybody home?"

Her greeting never came, and after a few moments of silence, I curiously walked out into the hallway to see why she was being so quiet. I was shocked to see her standing there white as a sheet and her eyes brimming with tears. This was very unlike her, and I felt a sense of dread as I quickly walked over to her and gently asked, "What's wrong, hon?"

She hung her head, lips quivering, and in a very small voice told me she had had an accident and her car was badly damaged. It had occurred only a few blocks from home, and she had abandoned it by the side of the road and walked home. She claimed she felt too shaken up to attempt driving any farther.

Of course, my first reaction was to look her over and ask her if she was all right, and she assured me that she was not physically hurt. I took her in my arms and tried to comfort her and calm her down. I was not particularly surprised that this accident had occurred. Perhaps subconsciously, I had been even waiting for it to happen.

I had noticed that lately her driving ability had seemed to be deteriorating, and she had become quite hesitant and indecisive in traffic. I had tried to tactfully speak to her about it, but she insisted she was fine and denied anything was wrong. She was quite defensive and annoyed with me for even suggesting there might possibly be a problem with her driving.

In retrospect, perhaps I should have been more adamant and forceful about it, but how do you tell an apparently healthy and relatively young woman in her sixties that she shouldn't drive anymore? There were other red flags as when she seemed to display minor confusion at understanding simple directions, or not grasping a joke as quickly as she used to.

I know now that I was in denial. I was deluding myself into thinking that there was really nothing particularly alarming about her behavior. After all, we all have our moments such as going into the next room for something and forgetting what it was we wanted when we get there. It was not difficult to accept her little lapses as fairly normal for our age. Stop being a worrisome old fool, nothing to really worry about, I would say to myself.

We, like most married couples, had quarreled on occasion, you know, kids, finances, etc, like I believe most everyone else usually has, but for the most part, we had been very compatible. Now it seemed I was in constant trouble with her, and nothing I did was right. I tried to ignore it when she would sulk for days at a time like a petulant teenager. I was confused and annoyed while I tried to fathom out what in the world I had done this time to set her off.

My patience was running thin, but I tried to contain my anger surmising that part of the problem was probably due to the fact that her father had passed away recently. I rationalized that she was going through a difficult period due to grief. In addition to missing him, she now also had the responsibility of consoling and caring for her widowed mother who was legally blind but fortunately lived nearby, so it was easy to reach her. Yes, I thought, this was certainly at least part of the problem.

Grandma Ann, as she was called by our children, was really a very nice lady. She and I had always been able to get along well, but she was also a very strong-minded woman who was used to having her own way. She was a typical Italian mother who felt her primary mission in this life was to feed the world. She loved to cook, particularly for her family.

Grandpa Ray, Terry's father, was a professional chef. When they worked in the kitchen together, it was their custom to fight constantly about how the cooking should be done.

"Ray, Ray," she would yell at him, "you're burning the meat!"

"Let me alone," he would shout back, "I know what I'm doing."

I can't imagine how they ever managed to do it, but every meal at their home was not only a true culinary delight but a picture to behold.

"Presentation is half the battle," they would say, smiling at each other. They were justifiably proud of their efforts, and the dinner was always delicious. The shouting was considered normal behavior for them and was soon completely forgotten. They loved to entertain, and an invitation to their home for dinner was something we all looked forward to.

Grandpa Ray was a sweet easygoing man who catered to Grandma's every whim. He and I were best buddies. We golfed together, went to football games, and just enjoyed each other's company. He loved it and would laugh when I would tell him, with a straight face, how much I hated him because he was so much better looking than me.

The truth was that he really was a very handsome man, and Grandma was very jealous when other women looked his way. When he died, she could not understand why everyone did not jump to fill her every desire as he so graciously used to do. She was a bit on the demanding side, although I doubt if she ever truly realized it.

Terry had always been so capable and independent that the idea of her needing any help from me never entered my mind. This accident caused a light bulb to go on in my brain, and I mentally chastised myself for not realizing that caring for her mother, while continuing to go to work, was putting quite a load on her. I can only guess that it was some misplaced sense of pride in her abilities that prevented her from asking for, or admitting, that she needed help from me or anyone else.

As I held her in my arms trying to soothe her, I was surprised to hear her say she did not want to drive anymore. I was aware that this was probably just the way she felt at the moment, and I felt certain that she would change her mind once she got over the shock of the accident. Oddly enough, it was my own sense of relief at hearing her say that she did not want to drive anymore that surprised me even more.

I began to realize that I must have been hiding my inner fears all along. My poor judgment could have caused her to be badly injured in an accident like the one that had just occurred or possibly injure someone else. I had had a wakeup call, and now that I was cognizant of my true feelings, I realized that this was perhaps a great opportunity for me to prevent her from continuing to drive, at least for a while, until she was hopefully herself again.

As I suspected she would do, she started to back down almost immediately.

"How can I take care of my mother if I don't drive?" she asked. "I have to drive even if I don't want to," she said, half choking with indecision.

I knew what she meant. There were doctor appointments that Grandma had to attend, shopping jaunts they both enjoyed, prescriptions that had to be picked up, and a million errands to be run. It was understandable that Terry did not want to give these things up. Not only were these outings fun for them, but also many of them were real necessities.

Yes, the accident had been a rude awakening for me, and I realized that I was going to have to step up to the plate and find a way to be more supportive. The problem was how to overcome that deep sense of independence that years of marriage had taught me Terry possessed. I feared she would refuse my help unless I could find a very diplomatic method of presenting my offer of assistance to her.

"Look," I said, "you're going to be without a car for a week or two while I get your car repaired for you. We could rent a car, but what for? How about letting me help you out for a short time or until you're feeling better about the accident and want to drive again. I'll drive you and your mom on your usual errands and take you wherever you need to go until you're ready to fly on your own again."

She looked up at me and said, "Do you really mean it? That would be wonderful."

"Sure," I said. I didn't want to sound too condescending and rouse any misgivings on her part, so I added a stipulation. "After all, it won't be forever. I'm enjoying my retirement too much. All I ask is that you work with me and try not to make any appointments on my golf days."

Saying it wouldn't be forever seemed to do the trick, and she half grudgingly and half gratefully accepted my offer to help.

"Okay, I guess it would be a big help if you would drive us around, but just for a while until the car is fixed and I am over this," she answered.

"That's what I said, just until you're over it. Let me know when you're ready to drive again and we'll talk."

Deep down I was already trying to think of what I would say when, and if, we ever had that talk. I was determined to find a way to keep her from driving no matter what. I decided to press my luck. Terry had taken over doing the household accounts for both ourselves and her mother. Being the family accountant and paying the bills were responsibilities that she seemed to enjoy doing and I believe gave her a certain sense of importance.

Because I was aware of this, I was not at all sure it was a chore she would be willing to surrender. I had noticed that she seemed to be laboring longer when she wrote out checks to pay our bills, but I had not thought much about it. Probably just a few extra bills from the department stores, I theorized.

I guess I shocked her when I said, "You have been pretty busy lately with your mom and all, why don't you let me give you a real vacation by going all the way for a while? I wouldn't mind taking over the household accounts just until you are your old self again. Relax and enjoy yourself with your mom for a while, you deserve it. Now that I am retired, it would give me something to do, and you can take over again anytime you want."

"You mean for my mom too?" she asked.

"Sure, why not."

I knew I would have no problem, having done my own books when I was in business, but I did not want her to feel I doubted her ability in any way.

"Besides, if I get into trouble I can always ask you for help, right?"

I guess the idea that she would still be needed was what she wanted to hear because after only a slight hesitation, she agreed, "For the time being of course," she said.

"Of course," I answered.

I guess I had been incredibly dense in not recognizing the stress she was under. In addition to the responsibilities she had taken on in order to care for her mother, I discovered things had not been going well in her job.

The company she worked for had an educational program that enabled her to attend college at night in order to attain an associate degree in accounting. She studied hard, and not only were we proud of her acquiring a sheepskin, but also the fact that she graduated as a straight A student. It is heartbreaking to realize that anyone with her prior mental ability could deteriorate into the poor lost soul she has become today. Alzheimer's has no respect for intelligence.

Shortly after she received her degree, they promoted her to assistant manager of the accounting department. It was a good job. She was content and was well thought of by both management and her coworkers.

An unfortunate situation developed that put her in an awkward position. It appeared that an office romance was developing involving Terry's immediate superior and one of the ladies in the office, both of whom were already married. They were not particularly discreet about their involvement, and some of the other ladies were offended by their blatant attitude.

They decided it was their moral duty to take some type of action and began to pressure Terry, as their superior, to do something about it. It was quite a difficult situation for Terry and posed quite a dilemma for her.

Naturally she did not relish going over the head of her superior, a man who had treated her well, nor did she appreciate being badgered by her coworkers. It was a damned-if-you-do and damned-if-you-don't situation.

In retrospect and knowing what I know now, I suspect she may also have been having trouble performing her duties at work. She surprised me when she told me of her problems at work and came to me for advice. I gave it some deep thought. Ordinarily, having been in management most of my life, I probably would have approached her problem at work differently had I not had these other concerns about her. I tried to weigh all the factors, and something inside me counseled caution. I decided that now was not a good time for her to enter into this type of dispute. I reasoned that she did not need any additional stress. She had enough on her plate.

Being older than she, I had naturally retired before her. I had been after her for quite some time to give notice to her employers and join me in retirement. The accident and the problems she had at work gave me additional incentive to press her into taking the plunge. I decided that it was to her advantage if I could remove her from this no-win situation. I took what I considered to be the easy way out for her and struck while the iron was hot.

"You don't need this type of aggravation at work, you have enough to do taking care of your mom. Think about it, wouldn't now be a great time to retire and live the good life with me, think of the fun we could have." I assured her she would love it.

"Can we get by if we both retire?" she asked.

"You know what we have as well as I," I answered.

She smiled up at me. It was the first smile she had given me since she had walked in the door, and I knew I was on the right track.

"Yeah, I guess we could," she said, and that resolved that. It had been easier than I thought with some degree of relief.

The following Monday, we rose out of bed, had breakfast, and I drove her to work. Although she still had some reservations, she shocked everyone by declaring that she was ready to join me in retirement.

"Why should he have all the fun?"

Everyone laughed, and this was her excuse for leaving. She gave her employer two weeks' notice that day, and I drove her to work and picked her up every day until her time was up. Her coworkers threw her a nice farewell party and wished her well with an abundance of hugs and tears. She did not comment on how she felt about retiring to me, nor did I question her, but I do believe she was feeling a good deal more relief than she wanted to admit.

I realized I had been a bit manipulative, but I was content that nothing I had done was self-serving. On the contrary, I suddenly found myself to be a chauffeur and package carrier for two women, Terry and her mom. I had Terry's car repaired, and when I suggested we sell it, I was stunned and relieved that there was absolutely none of the protest I had expected Terry to give me. The mold was set, and "Just for the time being!" became forever. To my relief, Terry has never driven again.

I was not particularly thrilled with my new role. It was not exactly what I had in mind for my retirement years, but I could not think of any other option if I wanted to keep her safe by her not driving. In a way, it was fun in the beginning. I would shake my head and woefully complain that I had become a slave to two evil, diabolical women who had absolutely no mercy on a poor exhausted old man.

"Poor Louis, he has it so tough," they would say, and then they would break up with laughter, which was exactly the effect I was looking for. I did manage to have quite a bit of fun with them, and I got a kick out of seeing how they enjoyed my feigned misery. Terry did seem more relaxed, and the concern I had felt for her well-being eased off a little. All in all I felt I had handled things fairly tactfully, and everything was working out pretty well.

I could not completely deny that things seemed to be different. She just was not the same fun-loving and capable Terry.

There were some things about her that just didn't seem right to me, and because of this, and with a great deal of effort, I managed to keep any anger or annoyance I was feeling in check. I discovered that for a hot-blooded Latin, I had found more self-control than I ever imagined I was capable of.

I continued to rationalize that this was just a phase she was going through due to her grief and that things would change back to normal eventually. The possibility of Alzheimer's did creep into my mind, but I quickly dismissed it as something that could not happen to us. Terry had always taken good care of herself and I believed to be in excellent health. Heck, I really didn't have things too bad. This was just a slight inconvenience that I would have to put up with for a while, no big deal. Once again I was confident that I had the ability to adjust to this slightly annoying situation. After all, I consoled myself, Terry and I still had our evenings out to go dancing with friends. I still had my golf days and lunches with the guys. Having the two ladies keep me busy and off the couch was probably a good thing for me as well as them.

It does not happen in all cases, but for many, denial is the first reaction, and it is easy to find excuses as I did. Many feel anger: Why is he or she doing this to me? Is he or she behaving this way deliberately just to annoy me?

The same question over and over again and she doesn't listen to my answer but keeps on asking. Man oh man, she does the dumbest things, and I have to watch her every minute. The reality is the patients have no control over their actions. Alzheimer's, nah, no way, not us, it's something else. Well, then again, perhaps it is.

Grandma Ann

I have a friend who greets each day in a novel way. Every morning before he gets out of bed, he rolls over, and in a very contrite voice, he says to his wife, "I'm sorry, honey."

Experience has taught him that it is a rare day when he does not do something wrong, at least in his wife's eyes. His philosophy is that he may as well try to blunt the effect of whatever transgression she may perceive he has performed. Getting the "I'm sorry, Hon" out of the way as soon as possible was usually good for a laugh from her, and at least they were starting the day off in a good mood.

I wondered if my starting the day off by taking a page out of his book might not be a good idea to try with Terry. She had always had a good sense of humor, but unfortunately she failed to see the humor in it, and it did not work for me. The moodiness and sulking, although it had lessened, still continued no matter how hard I tried to be agreeable.

I started to take over most of the responsibilities that had been Terry's as I had volunteered to do. Paying the bills and taking care of the paperwork offered no problem to me and really took very little of my time. I was puzzled with the fact that Terry had found it difficult and had needed to labor over it the way she did. She had always been so capable.

Terry had insisted that all decisions concerning her mother's well-being and health were her responsibility. This was certainly understandable to me. As a loving daughter, she would naturally feel that no one else could care for her mother as well as she could.

As promised, I started to drive them to the various doctor's appointments that Grandma was periodically required to attend. Terry asked me if I would mind coming in with them and listening to everything the doctor had to say. In view of Terry's attitude about being in charge of her mom's well-being, the request mildly surprised me. I said nothing but nodded my head in agreement.

I noticed that after the visits, Terry would want to discuss what the doctor had said with me. I considered this to be perfectly normal in the beginning, but as we talked, I began to suspect from some of her comments and questions that she was having difficulty grasping what the doctor's instructions were and was looking for clarification from me. Even after I would go over what the doctor had said to her, when it actually came time to perform these instructions, she would ask for my assistance. I began to realize that this was because she was becoming quite unsure of herself.

Terry and I had, for the most part, always had what I considered a better than average relationship in our marriage. We had, without ever really discussing, or probably even realizing it, adopted and ceded to each other the responsibilities for those tasks for which each seemed to be better qualified. For example, she was the better cook, and I was better at yard work. Of course, as I mentioned, we had our disputes, but we were both comfortable in the marital roles we had chosen for ourselves. I suppose I egotistically thought it was really I who was in charge and that it was very nice of me to allow her to feel she was in charge of certain aspects of our marriage.

As I grew older and wiser, I had to laugh at myself when I realized she was playing the same game with me. I suspect, although we never spoke of it, that she had figured it all out too. It had worked well though because our little game had caused our marriage to evolve into a fairly equal partnership, and as partners do, we discussed problems, sometimes we argued, but we were usually able to reach an agreeable compromise that we could both live with on most issues. She was smart, and I appreciated her input on various issues. She in turn, I am sure, respected my thinking also.

I suddenly found myself making all the decisions. I had hoped that by trying to understand Terry's problems, and by my making every effort to give her any assistance she seemed to need, things would start to go back to the way they used to be. Instead I was now truly in charge and making all the decisions on my own. The truth was that I missed my old partner's input. It was great, I now admitted, to have someone to bounce your thinking off. As the old saying goes, "Be careful what you wish for, you might just get it."

As I had mentioned, the sulking still continued and would often occur, for no apparent reason, in the presence of other family members and friends. It was not only embarrassing to me but to everyone else who witnessed it. Terry had always been good company and fun to be with, but now her personality change was causing heads to turn.

I tried to make light of it, but it took a good deal of patience on my part not to take issue with her right on the spot when this occurred. The looks that some of my friends gave me left me with no doubt as to what they were thinking when they looked at me. What happened to Lou, has he become a wimp? I had to swallow hard, and actually I did not quite understand my own restraint. I was not exactly noted for my patience. What was holding me back? I wondered.

A close friend of mine found the courage to ask, "What did you ever do to make her so mad at you all the time?"

He thought it was hilarious when I answered truthfully, "I haven't got a clue."

Personally I didn't think it was so funny, but I guess I could see why he would. There were periods of time when she would be fine. She would almost be her old self. She seemed more alert, and everything appeared normal again. Anyone meeting her for the first time would not be aware anything was wrong. She would be good for days and suddenly go off the deep end again. It was very confusing.

Grandma Ann had eventually come to live with us after Grandpa Ray had passed away. It was difficult for her to give up her own little condo with all its wonderful memories of good times with Grandpa Ray and the rest of the family. It was a beautiful little two-bath, two-bedroom condo whose screened-in porch overlooked the seventh green of a very nice private golf course. It was tastefully decorated with many of the lovely cherished possessions they had acquired over a lifetime.

She was quite healthy and sharp as a tack mentally, but because of her poor eyesight and the fact that she also had to wear hearing aids, she needed quite a bit of help. In addition to these afflictions, she had a terrible phobia about being left alone. She really did not want to leave her condo, but all of these formidable problems had to be addressed somehow.

We suggested various options to her and investigated those that seemed to interest her. She finally decided that it would be best if we hired a woman who had been recommended to us through our church. We were told the woman was quite experienced in care giving and understood that Grandma would be quite dependent on her because of her disabilities. She assured us that she could handle things, and she seemed to be the perfect person to move in with Grandma and tend to her needs. We gave her a try.

Terry and I would visit Grandma at her condo almost every day to see how things were going, but it soon became evident, at least to me, that Grandma was not happy with this arrangement.

I asked Grandma what was wrong, and she confided in me that the woman, although capable, was very quiet and reserved. Grandma wanted a companion, someone she could talk to, gossip with, and laugh with. The woman was very devout, and when she was not caring for Grandma, she spent her time praying and watching religious programs on TV. There was, of course, nothing wrong with this, I would never criticize someone for their faith, but she was not supplying the companionship that Grandma craved. It was not working, and I had to, as gently as possible, let her go.

Surrendering our privacy was not an easy decision for us to make, but after much soul-searching, we knew that it was just about our only viable option. Grandma resisted but we finally convinced her that it would probably be best for her, and us, if she would come and live with us.

Originally Terry and I had lived in a similar condo in the same complex that Grandma lived in, more about that later, but as our family grew with the advent of grandchildren, we decided to build a larger home in order to be able to accommodate everyone for family gatherings. We did not sell our condo but decided to keep it and rent it out as an investment.

Our home was a split-plan ranch with a secluded screened-in swimming pool that eventually all our grandchildren learned to swim in. Our bedroom and bath was on one side of the house, and the other side contained two bedrooms and a bath.

There was a sliding door that when closed separated that part of the house from the living quarters. Grandma would have the privacy of her own little apartment with her own private bath. There was a large family room with a fireplace next to the living room. The dining room was just off the eat-in kitchen and was very convenient for family parties. It was a nicely designed and comfortable home.

It should have been a perfect situation, and we tried hard to make Grandma feel welcome, but it soon became painfully apparent that we had very different interests. My own chauvinistic theory was that the ladies of Grandma's generation were primarily women whose duties had consisted of raising children, doing the cooking, keeping the house clean and neat, and taking care of their husbands. Their conversation usually ran toward minding each other's business, or to put it bluntly, they loved to gossip or discuss how they suffered with their various ailments.

In the beginning, we managed some small amount of conversation about family members and what was new with them, but that topic would soon run out. Grandma would prattle on about some juicy piece of gossip that had occurred twenty years ago. Some of it was funny, but most of it we had heard many times before, and we could not help but tire of hearing the same stories over and over. She, conversely, was not particularly interested in much that we had to say about current topics. The most animated conversation we would have on any given day was deciding what we were going to prepare for dinner that night.

As I mentioned, Terry was pretty good most of the time, but her mood changes and sulking were a source of concern for her mother. In spite of the many red flags that were waving at me, I still stubbornly fought against believing anything was really wrong.

I had come to the incorrect conclusion that my best defense against my wife's behavior, short of murder or divorce, was to ignore her. Grandma would sit in the corner of the couch and snooze during these sessions in order to escape the deafening silence when Terry would sulk. Terry and her mother had always gotten along well, but now, with her personality change, she was unwittingly confusing and hurting her mother.

"What's wrong with Teresa, Lou?" Grandma would ask.

"I guess she misses Grandpa and going to work," I would answer.

"You really think that's it?"

"Sure, she'll get over it soon, you'll see." I would try to soothe her.

"I don't know, I don't know," she would doubtfully say and shake her head.

I hated to see the old lady subjected to these displays of temperament from her daughter. I would try to assure her that all was well with Terry, but I was at last beginning to have difficulty suppressing my own growing suspicions.

Grandma's questions began to worry me. Was Grandma seeing more than I was? Perhaps my assessment of Terry's problems was not exactly accurate. Could it be that maybe something really was wrong?

Just when my suspicions would begin to peak, Terry would have a few of her good days and behave perfectly normal. She would be pleasant, behave intelligently, and seem to have no problem performing simple everyday tasks. When this would occur, it would send me back the other way, and I would again resist the idea that there was anything of a medical nature that could be wrong with her.

Perhaps she was just going through some kind of hormonal phase similar to menopause. All would return to normal in time. I was grasping at straws. Although I had made many adjustments and struggled for patience, I found myself shamefully trying to avoid her company. I was much less in a hurry to return home when I had completed an errand or was through playing golf. I worried about my masculinity. Was I allowing myself to turn into a henpecked Caspar Milktoast whose only response to his difficult wife was "Yes, dear"?

After a few days of one of her sulking moods, I tried asking her what the problem was.

"What's wrong, Terry," I asked.

She gave me a blank stare and said, "Nothing is wrong with me, I was wondering what I did to make you so angry. Why aren't you talking to me?"

Her answer made me blink in confusion. "You started sulking and stopped talking to me," I would say.

"No I didn't. It's not me who's sulking, it's you, everything is fine with me."

She evidently had no recollection of going off into one of her moods. I would shake my head in frustration. Things were not working out well with Grandma, and no one was content. Grandma worried about Terry, and Terry was constantly annoyed with Grandma. I was caught in the middle trying to play the role of peacemaker. Grandma would retreat to the couch and close her eyes. I knew something had to be done.

I caught Terry in one of her better moods and decided to broach a subject that had begun to form in my mind. It was a delicate subject, and I had been waiting to find the proper moment to approach it. I thought this might be that moment.

"Your mom's asleep in the corner of the couch again," I commented.

"Yeah," Terry answered. "She sure doesn't act like my old mom."

I let that slide.

"You know, hard as we try, I don't think she is very happy living with us. Aside from talking about family, food, and our little excursions, we don't seem to have much in the way of common interests. I know she misses your father a lot, but we just don't seem able to fill the void regardless of our attempts to entertain her."

She agreed with me again. "You're right, but I don't know what to do about it."

We had a close friend who had been through a similar problem with her mother. After some very serious thought, she and her husband finally convinced themselves that placing her mom in an assisted-living facility might be better for all concerned. Surprisingly her mom adjusted in a relatively short time, and things worked out quite well for them. In view of the difficulty Terry and Grandma were having with each other, it was an alternative that I had given some thought to. I had hesitated and was naturally concerned over what Terry's reaction might be if I expressed my thinking to her.

Terry's momentary good mood offered me an opportunity to hesitantly introduce my thoughts to her.

I decided to take the bull by the horns and speak up while she was in a mood where there was at least a small possibility that she might be receptive.

"Your mother is going to die in the corner of that couch if we don't find something to keep her stimulated."

Terry's eyes began to tear up. "What do you have in mind?" she asked.

Here goes nothing, I thought to myself.

"I hate to say this, but wouldn't she be happier with people her own age that have similar interests? We love her, and she loves us, but the truth is that except for our little outings she is bored stiff."

Terry just sat there without answering.

I continued on, "Things seem to have worked out very well for our friend. Her mom seems to have adapted to the assisted-living facility quite easily, and they tell us she is very happy. Don't you think it might be something we should at least look into?"

Terry continued to shake her head. "I couldn't do it, and even if I could, she would never go for it."

I shifted gears. "I don't believe it is something we are ever really going to do," I said. "I just think that for her sake we should at least explore the possibility. It will be more of an exercise for us to satisfy ourselves that this was an option we took the time to look into and consider. We owe it to her, and ourselves, to at least investigate the possibility that there might be a better way of life for her out there."

"Oh god! Oh my god! I don't know, I don't know," she moaned.

"It's just a thought, something for us to do," I hedged. "We don't have to actually do anything or say anything to

Grandma. I'm just curious to see what these places are like in the event it becomes something we are someday forced to do. We are not getting any younger, and I am wondering what would happen to Grandma if one of us became ill. I don't want to be morbid, but some of our friends that were younger than we are have already passed on."

Terry looked up at me, and I could see that I had struck a nerve and had her attention. I suppose at this point I appear to be a selfish son-in-law who wants to get rid of his mother-in-law. This was not the case at all. I really loved the old lady, and in a way it was her well-being that I was thinking of. I had not told Terry all that was on my mind. As I mentioned earlier, Terry had always been a loving and considerate daughter, but now she seemed constantly annoyed with her mom. They were curt in their conversations with each other, and although they did not fight or really argue, there was a very thick feeling of tension in the air. Occasionally they would relax and bury the hatchet recalling some old memory that would cause them to chat normally for a while. Inevitably Terry would fall back into one of her quiet sulking moods, and Grandma would look at me in puzzlement and ask again, "What's wrong with Teresa, Lou?"

"I don't know, Grandma, she seems okay most of the time. I think she will get over it eventually. Let's give it some more time and see what happens."

I honestly believed it would be best for all of us if they did not have to live together. I hoped it would ease the pressure. I suspected Terry was feeling guilty over her mother and that she would perhaps return to normal if I could make that go away.

I spoke to our friends about how her mother was doing in the ALF while Terry sat and listened. I asked for their advice and how they liked the place she was in. I looked in the yellow pages for those facilities that were closest to us, and with a little urging, Terry agreed to visit a few of the facilities with me.

I am not sure what we were expecting, but the stigmatized image of an old folk's home with its senile and uncared for residents was obviously no longer valid. We were surprisingly pleased by what we discovered. The places we checked out were clean and bright, and the food we saw appeared to be tasty and nutritious. The residents seemed content, and best of all, they were in approximately the same age group as Grandma.

Hopefully their interests would be similar, and she would have people to converse with, which was just what Grandma needed. There were also activities and entertainment to keep them occupied. Each resident lived in a nicely decorated room with their own private bathroom. We spoke to a few of the residents, and the majority of them appeared to be quite content. Of course, there were a few malcontents, but it was not difficult to discern that they were individuals that nothing or no one could ever completely satisfy. There could be no doubt that we were both impressed with what we had seen, but we were also torn with guilt and probably more confused than ever.

We could see where living in an ALF environment might well be the best thing for her, and yes, for us too. Besides our own sense of guilt, there was also the nagging fear of what the rest of Terry's family would think if we put Grandma in a so-called old folk's home.

We agonized with indecision. The facility we liked best was the same one our friends' mother was in and only about two miles from where we lived. We would be able to visit her often, so she would hopefully not feel deserted. Our biggest problem was that we dreaded broaching the idea with her and feared what her reaction would be. We knew that it would be natural for a woman her age to be frightened of such a drastic change, and it was something that we had carefully taken into consideration.

We searched our conscience, and after much discussion, we both honestly felt that we should at least attempt to offer her what we honestly believed would be a better and happier lifestyle. I finally decided that the time had come for me to broach the subject with Grandma if the opportunity presented itself.

Terry was having one of her better days, and one evening, in the course of conversation at dinner, I brought up the subject of how well our friends' mother was doing in her ALF. Terry and I spoke about how much she enjoyed the entertainment and the activities and how she had made many new friends to converse with. Grandma listened with interest, nodding her head and asking questions, but when we suggested that she too might be happier with people her own age to talk to, she responded with a resounding "No, it wouldn't be for me."

We would bring the subject up every so often but to no avail. "Sounds nice," she would say, "but it's not for me." "It's not for me" was her consistent answer.

One evening I mentioned that we were going to meet our friends at the assisted living facility to pick up her mother and then we were going out for lunch afterward. Grandma had met our friends' mother on a few previous occasions before she went into the ALF, and I casually told Grandma she was welcome to come along if she wished. Going out to lunch was one of Grandma's favorite pastimes, and she readily accepted the invitation.

We met our friends at the appointed time and went into the ALF to visit with her mother for a short time before we all went to lunch. We had filled our friends in on what we were up to, and they suggested that we take a tour of the facility. In the process of the tour, Grandma stopped and visited with some of the resident ladies. She found them quite sociable, and we could see she was enjoying herself.

One lecherous old guy came over and flirted with her, telling her, with a little wink, that he thought she had a nice figure. She feigned annoyance at his compliment, but she told everyone she knew about it, and it was obvious that she enjoyed the flattery. We all had a pleasant lunch, and when we returned home that evening, we asked Grandma what she thought of the place.

"It was nicer than I thought it would be," she said, "but it wouldn't be for me."

"You're probably right, too much talking going on all the time, it would drive me crazy," I said.

She looked at me like I was crazy. Talking, as I well knew, was her favorite pastime. I think she was waiting for me to try and push her, and she was actually surprised at my comment. I knew that pushing her would only make her resist more.

"Actually I enjoyed talking to those ladies," she admitted defensively.

"You did?" I answered, pretending to be amazed. "Well, if you ever want to give it a try for a few days to see if you really like it, you know you can move back in with us anytime you want. Come to think of it, you really wouldn't have a thing to lose, and you could look at it like you were taking a little vacation. Could be a pleasant change for you."

She grew quiet, and I could hear the wheels turning in her head. We talked about it on and off, and after a few days of falling asleep with boredom on the couch, she came to me and said, "I'm only doing this to please you, but I'm ready to give it a try. You promise I can come back if I don't like it, right?"

"Of course," I said.

The big day came. She was all packed, and her knees were getting weaker by the moment. She repeatedly recited her favorite adages when things were not going the way she wanted: "It's doomsday" and "I know this is curtains for me."

We too had serious misgiving about our decision as she very deftly laid a beautiful guilt trip on us. Her words went through us like a knife. We were close to picking up the phone and calling the whole thing off. We drove the short distance to the facility and got her settled in her room. Several of the ladies came over and welcomed her, and this seemed to relax her as we chatted away the afternoon with them.

Dinner was about to be served, and it was time for us to leave. Our fingers were crossed as we kissed her good-bye, but thankfully there were no tears from Grandma. We drove home slowly, and I noticed that Terry took out a hanky and wiped her eyes. In all honesty, although I felt I had done what was best for all concerned, I found I had to wipe my eyes too.

I am not exaggerating when I tell you that within two weeks I don't think we could have coerced her into coming back to live with us at gunpoint. She was filled with gossip every time we visited her, and we were given a complete rundown on the life history of every resident living there. The owners jokingly told us that they were no longer hesitant to go on vacation because Grandma was now in complete charge and running the place.

I am well aware that things do not always work out this well in many cases, but for Grandma, it was obviously the correct decision. She was happy and animated again, and any sense of guilt we may have felt rapidly disappeared. In a way it was a good lesson for me. The thought ran through my mind that the day could possibly come when I honestly could no longer take care of myself or Terry. If the realization ever presents itself that either of us would be better cared for elsewhere, then I hope this experience will help me to do what is right for us and ease the pain I know I will feel.

There had been some dissention, as we had feared there might be, from some of Grandma's siblings. They sent a delegation down from New York to check up on their poor sister who had been deserted and forced into a terrible institution by an unfeeling daughter and son-in-law. I suspect they had visions of their sister sitting in the corner of a dingy room with a bowl of gruel on a table before her. A muscular matron would be standing over her forcing her to eat. Their demeanor was very cool, and

Terry was obviously hurt. I too felt very uncomfortable and had the impression that they were ready to take her back with them.

We took them over to the ALF to visit Grandma, and they were soon very impressed with the cleanliness and cheerful ambiance of the place. It was obvious to them how content and alive she was compared to the last time they had seen her when she had lived with us.

They admitted they had had some serious misgivings over what we had done with Grandma, but then to our relief they smiled and said the words we had hoped and prayed they would: "You made the right decision."

Saying Good-Bye
To Grandma

Grandma was pretty well settled in and was definitely content with her new environment in the ALF. Terry did seem to be a little less tense now, and I was spending less time in the doghouse. I surmised that it was because she was more at ease now that she had been relieved from a good portion of her care giving responsibilities. I believe she was also was quite content with the knowledge that her mother was being well taken care of.

Terry and I continued to run errands for Grandma. We would drive her to her many doctor appointments and visited her several times a week as did her grandchildren whenever they got the chance. I picked my times to visit and only took Terry to visit when she was in one of her better moods. I tried hard to protect Grandma from seeing her when she was in one of her sulking moods.

Grandma always had a list waiting for us when we came, and we would shop for whatever she asked for. Her toiletries were the most difficult things to please her with. Things always seemed to be the wrong brand, the wrong size, or the wrong color, and we were constantly exchanging things. This could become quite frustrating, and I am afraid I did not always do it with the utmost of grace. It was a standing joke among her grandchildren, all of whom adored her, that you must keep the receipt for anything you purchased for Grandma. You were almost certain to have to exchange it.

I don't know how she did it, but it was unbelievable the amount of things she could find for me to do. Terry was becoming increasingly dependent on me, and along with Grandma's demands, I was getting snowed under. Fortunately my daughter and daughter-in-law suspected about what was happening to me and offered to help by running some of Grandma's errands for me. They had no idea what they were letting themselves in for.

It did not take long for them to also become amazed at how busy Grandma could keep all three of us. I found it quite humorous watching the awestruck expressions on their faces when they spoke of it to others, and I had difficulty suppressing my laughter. I suspect they had not really believed us when they overheard Terry and I talking about how busy Grandma was keeping us. Now they knew.

"Why didn't you say something sooner?" they admonished me.

"I don't think you would have believed me," I answered.

Grandma was as good-hearted a person as anyone I had ever known, but was noted by the family for sometimes speaking with very little tactfulness. Sometimes when we visited her, she would question me about Terry's "condition" in front of Terry as though Terry was not there. This, of course, annoyed Terry, and she would adamantly insist that she was fine. I would nod my head in agreement with Terry and try to stave off any confrontation between the two women.

I managed to get Grandma alone, and I asked her to please not do that anymore. I guess she was a bit hurt, but she did stop doing it. The truth was that too many red flags were beginning to appear that I too could no longer overlook. My own concerns for Terry were increasing every day.

Grandma had a favorite joke that she loved to tell. It was about a man who had buried three wives, two of whom had died of food poisoning and one from a fractured skull. When asked how come the last one died of a fractured skull, he answered, "She wouldn't eat the mushrooms." Grandma laughed louder than anyone at her own joke, and although we had all heard it many times before, we all could not help but to laugh too.

Grandma knew she was keeping me quite busy, and to her credit, she was quite grateful and would often thank me for all I was doing. She would apologize for all the, as she put it, "extra work" she was causing me. I would kid her that I wouldn't have to do so much if she would only eat her mushrooms. She had a sense of humor, and when I teased her like this, she would laugh along with me. She knew I was only fooling with her, but I guess she wasn't completely sure because the really humorous part of this story is that, although she had always loved them, I don't believe she ever ate mushrooms again for the rest of her life.

It had been my hope that I could protect Grandma from her suspicions that something might be wrong with Terry. I felt that if Terry really did have a problem that it was not something that Grandma needed to know, and worry about, at her age. In spite of my best efforts, Grandma was becoming increasingly suspicious. I tried to assure her that things would probably improve, but she would look at me very doubtfully and shake her head. She really was too smart to fool.

She became less and less secure with Terry's judgment and started to turn to me more and more for direction and anything she needed help with. Grandma and I became very close in those years, and no matter what the problem was, or what decision had to be made, her response was always "Ask my son-in-law."

Her dependency and confidence in me was very flattering, and without my realizing it at the time, I had slowly fallen into the role of Grandma's caregiver. It was a pretty good initiation into what the future held in store for me as Terry's caregiver.

Grandma was very content at the ALF for many years and made many close friends. Occasionally she would find something to complain about, and I would tease her by asking her if she wanted to come back and live with us, or perhaps she would like me to look for another place for her to stay. She would pretend to consider my offer, but she always declined. "I'll just have to make the best of it," she would bravely say, and then emit a long sigh of resignation. The complaints would stop, and it was obvious that she really was happy and wanted to stay right where she was.

Grandma passed on at the ripe old age of ninety-three and was mentally alert right up until the last week or two of her life. It was only the medication that they were giving her, in order to keep her comfortable, that finally caused her mind to wander.

It was interesting to note that no one on either side of Terry's family had ever showed any signs of dementia and lived to a ripe old age. The really confusing thing was that, regardless of this, it was not only she who had dementia, but her brother eventually contracted it too.

One day as Grandma lay in her hospital bed, and was approaching the end, she asked me to come closer because she wanted to whisper something in my ear.

"Promise me you'll take care of Terry, Lou," she said.

I had to pause and swallow the lump that suddenly appeared in my throat before I could answer.

"I will, Grandma, I promise you I will," I answered.

Even in her drug-induced dreams, Grandma was still feeding people, and the last words I can remember hearing her proudly say to her imaginary guests were, "Of course we have ice cream." She was a good old gal, and I really miss her.

The First Diagnosis

Terry's forgetfulness and odd behavior was becoming more and more noticeable. She would often ask the same question over and over again. At first I would snap back at her and answer her with a "I just told you that, pay attention, will you?" She would look bewildered and in a little while ask the same question again.

I finally realized that she just didn't remember asking the question before. It was not an easy thing to do, but I learned to either change the subject or answer the question as often as she asked it. Snapping at her accomplished nothing except to hurt her feelings and make me hate myself for doing it. Yes, the warning lights were beginning to shine brighter in my mind, and I could no longer stubbornly ignore them. There was no one thing in itself that was particularly alarming to me in my denial-prone mind. After all, as I have said before, we all have our moods and forgetful moments. Sadly I began to notice that when we were in a social atmosphere, family and friends would occasionally exchange inquisitive looks over something she said or did.

I tried to tactfully ask her if she felt everything was all right and perhaps gently mention something odd I had noticed in her behavior. She would deny anything was wrong and walk off in a huff. I had reached the point where I knew something had to be done, if for no other reasons than to put my own mind at ease. The question was, how do I handle this without frightening her or sending her off in one of her moods?

My dilemma was solved unexpectedly but unfortunately in a way that was absolutely heartrending to me. I was enjoying watching a little TV when I realized I had not seen Terry for a while. I called out her name, and when I received no answer, I got up and started to walk around the house to see where she was, just to make sure she was okay. I found her sitting quietly on the bed in our bedroom. Her lips were quivering, and she was close to tears.

I sat down next to her and as gently as I could I asked her, "What's wrong, hon, what can I do to help?"

She shook her head and said, "I'm just being silly," and then in a more toxic tone of voice, "Just forget it."

The tears in her eyes made me press the issue.

"No, I won't forget it," I said forcibly. "Something is bothering you, and I want to know what it is."

She hung her head, and the tears began to cascade down her cheeks. In a small voice that was little more than a whisper, she confessed her fears to me, "I'm worried that maybe something really is wrong with me."

Terry had always been a proud and somewhat private person who was not prone to complaining or admitting to any frailty. Her admission surprised me, and I realized for the first time that she was more aware of the changes in her behavior than I had thought. Behind her sulking, I suddenly realized, was a very frightened lady.

She too had been in denial for so long and insistent that nothing was wrong with her that this sudden reversal caught me off guard. I was at a loss for words for the moment. I wondered what she must be going through mentally and emotionally as these thoughts passed through her mind. I did not respond immediately. It was a very bad moment for me as well as her, and I was afraid to talk for fear my voice would break. I put my arm around her and took her hand in mind. She lay her head on my shoulder as she wept, and I put my other arm around her, hugging her to me. I too was filled with emotion as I tried to console her.

Finally I was able to speak, "Let me make an appointment for you with the doctor," I coaxed. "I'm sure there is nothing seriously wrong with you," I fibbed, "perhaps a vitamin deficiency or even a mild stroke at worse. You're due for a checkup anyhow, so let's kill two birds with one stone and see what the doctor has to say."

I thought I would run into some degree of stubborn resistance, but she quickly agreed.

"Maybe that isn't a bad idea," she answered, and there was actually a note of relief in her voice.

I quickly looked up the doctor's number and walked over to the phone with determination. I set up an appointment before she could change her mind. She had not been too receptive to my cornball humor lately, but I decided to see if I could ease her concern with a little bit of kidding. She was sixty-four years old at the time.

"I'm glad you're going in for a checkup because lately I have become a grouchy old bear married to a grouchy old tigress. I was thinking about putting an ad in the paper to see if I can swap you in for two thirty-year-olds."

My fingers were crossed and I was relieved when she started to laugh, "What would you do with two thirty-year-olds?" she kidded back.

"I believe I would think of something," I answered.

We were both laughing now, and it felt good. Actually we laughed a lot harder than that little bit of nonsense warranted. I guess, to some extent, it was because we were relieved that the fears we had both kept hidden inside us for so long were out in the open now. It was surprising how quickly her moods could change from tears to laughter. We got a lot of mileage out of that little bit of nonsense through the years that followed. Whenever she would get depressed and start to sulk, I would threaten to put the ad back in the newspaper. Most of the time, it worked, and she would laugh. Later on, even our friends picked up on it and would occasionally ask if I was getting any response to my ad. I would shake my head sadly to everyone's amusement.

When the day came for the doctor's appointment, I took the nurse aside and told her I wanted to speak to the doctor when she had completed Terry's physical examination. I knew my wife well enough to know what a private person she was, and I feared that she would hold back mentioning anything to the doctor about our concerns.

The doctor completed her examination, and I was called in as I had requested. The doctor smiled and told me Terry was in excellent physical condition. It was then that I tried to explain my concerns about Terry's confusion and behavior. Terry did not add much to what I said except to interject occasionally with comments such as, "Oh, it's really not that bad" or "I think he's exaggerating." She was still defending herself regardless of her own fears.

Anyone who has been an Alzheimer's caregiver will tell you how amazingly the afflicted one can rise to the occasion and appear to be perfectly normal in company. I have told you how some days were better than others, and on this particular day, she seemed quite alert and lucid. She certainly did not do or say anything that would alarm the doctor. I felt frustrated and embarrassed as Terry put on her act. I knew I must have appeared to be a worrisome old fool to the doctor.

The doctor listened to me politely nodding her head from time to time as doctors do and asked Terry a few simple questions, which she was able to answer. The doctor said that she saw nothing to be worried about and that Terry was probably just suffering from a slight case of depression. The doctor wrote out a prescription for an antidepressant and smiled reassuringly at me.

I had mixed emotions. On the one hand, I was happy with the doctor's diagnosis, but on the other hand, I knew the doctor had caught her on a good day and that her behavior on this day was far from her usual behavior at home. I could see no other option but to go along with the doctor's appraisal, at least for the time being.

The antidepressant did seem to help in that I was spending even less time in the doghouse and I no longer saw any signs of quivering lips or tears. Now that the sulking was abating to some extent, her sense of humor also seemed to improve. She still was not the old Terry, but the medication did do its job, and she was a lot calmer. I wondered if the doctor's diagnosis really was correct. Was I seeing more than was really there? Was she really not that bad?

I desperately wanted to believe she was okay. I wondered if my original theory that it was just the pressure of caring for her mother and the loss of her father that were the real culprits. These things along with the trouble at work that had caused her so much aggravation were enough to drive anyone up a wall. Sure, I rationalized, she was going to be okay. In retrospect, I doubt that I truly believed a word I was saying to myself.

The Second Diagnosis

I had suffered from a heart attack a few years back but had recovered nicely with the aid of the medication my cardiologist had prescribed and by changing and watching my diet. I believe that it is because I did as I was instructed by my doctors that my heart had checked out fine at all of my future physicals and I am still here and feeling good. One of the doctors claimed there was nothing like surviving a heart attack to make someone start taking care of themselves.

The hospital and cardiologist, both of which I had developed a good deal of confidence in, decided they would no longer accept the HMO to which Terry and I had belonged for many years. They claimed our present HMO was restricting them from giving proper care to their patients, and they would no longer use them. In order to retain these doctors, I had no choice but to switch Terry and me to a new HMO.

I did some investigating, and after a little research, I found a new HMO that was acceptable to my old doctors.

The truth was that neither Terry nor I were particularly fond of her original doctor, and it seemed a good time for her to switch. For this reason, Terry did not offer any resistance when I suggested we try finding a new doctor for her.

Actually I had switched doctors a while ago, and my first thought was to ask my doctor if he would consider accepting Terry as a new patient. He advised me that he was really not taking on any new patients, but he would accept Terry as a favor to me. He hesitated for a moment and then suggested another doctor who was a female internist. She worked in the same building as he, which was very convenient for me. He recommended her highly, and because Terry actually preferred a female doctor, we decided to take his advice, and we put our trust in her.

The new doctor insisted that she give Terry a complete physical in order to come up with her own conclusions. I liked this and was pleased with her apparent thoroughness. Once again I requested that I be allowed to speak to the doctor after Terry's physical was completed. After the usual waiting period, I was led into the examination room where I was able to describe Terry's behavior to the doctor and express my concerns. This time Terry did not say anything at all. She just sat there expressionless and quietly listening to what I had to say. I felt the dementia had noticeably progressed, and because Terry just sat there without any protest, I wondered if my suspicions would be confirmed this time. I prayed that I would be told again that there was really nothing to worry about, but I had the worrisome premonition that this time such would not be the case.

The doctor asked Terry a few questions very much like the ones the other doctor had asked, but this time I noticed that Terry had quite a bit more difficulty in answering some of them.

"It appears that Terry is displaying some degree of confusion and forgetfulness. She seems to be in perfect health physically, but I am concerned with her symptoms of dementia. I believe it would be best for Terry to see a neurologist for a more thorough examination," she said.

Terry looked over at me, showing no emotion at all. It was not one of her good days, and I was not sure she understood exactly what was happening. I knew she was looking for direction from me.

"Let's do as the doctor says, Hon," I gently urged.

Terry took a moment, and then she hesitantly nodded her head in agreement. The doctor wasted no time and immediately had her nurse arrange for an appointment with the neurologist the following week.

The neurologist was very pleasant and quickly put us both at ease. He told Terry he was going to ask her a few questions and not to worry if she could not answer some of them.

"It's not really a test," he said. "It's just a little game to see if we can find out if you have some small problem that we might be able to fix. I am going to give you five words to remember, and every so often, as we talk, I am going to ask you to tell me what those words were."

This all occurred some time ago, and I don't recall exactly what the words were, but they were simple words such as *dog*, *mother*, *house*, *car*, etc.

He asked easy questions at first.

"Are you married?"

She answered, "Yes," and then looked over at me as if to ask if that was right.

"Can you tell me for how long?"

She looked to me again for help, but the doctor shook his head at me, and I understood that I was to remain silent.

She struggled for a moment before she answered, "I don't remember."

He continued to ask simple questions.

"Do you have any children? How many? How many grandchildren?"

These were all questions she should easily have known, but she could not answer many of them. I wanted desperately to help her, and every question she should have known but could not answer went through me like a knife in my side. Periodically he would ask her to repeat the five words he had given her to remember. She could not remember more than one or two words at a time. If she answered a question correctly, he would praise her, and if she could not answer correctly, he assured her that it was all right. This would usually produce a bland smile from her.

The neurologist suggested that we submit her to an MRI and a few other tests in order to rule out a few of the possibilities that could be the cause of her problems. I readily agreed. There was no comment from Terry. An appointment was made for the MRI, and although I was concerned about how Terry would withstand the confining aspects of the test, she went through it with no difficulty at all.

In a few days, the doctor had the results of the MRI. His nurse phoned us to set up an appointment with the doctor so that he could explain what the MRI had revealed to us in person. The doctor explained that the MRI had shown that she had experienced a few minor strokes, which, he assured us, was perfectly normal for a woman her age. He then added that nothing of a serious nature, such as a brain tumor or an aneurism, had been detected.

I waited with dread for the other shoe to drop. In view of the difficulty she had shown in answering his questions, I suspected there was more to come, and it was not going to be good news. I wondered how Terry would react and what I could do, or say, to console her if my suspicions and fears were valid.

The doctor explained that at this point in time the only true way of determining if someone had Alzheimer's was to perform an autopsy after the patient had expired. He went on to say that the only way they could determine anything was by the process of elimination. In view of her obvious dementia, and the lack of anything else that could explain her problem, he believed she was in the early stages of Alzheimer's.

Terry and I had never spoken the word *Alzheimer's* to each other, although I am sure she had thought of it as I had. I guess it was a word neither of us had wanted to be the first to utter. Oddly she showed no reaction at all, it was as though she had not heard him. He took her hand and very kindly and gently assured her that she had done nothing wrong and that she was in no way to blame for her illness. This time she looked up at him and gave him one of her big dazzling smiles, still no comment from her.

The doctor and I exchanged glances, and I believe he might have been as amazed as I was at her reaction. I suspect he was used to seeing some tears and possibly even some hysteria, but she showed no emotion at all.

He went on to explain that there were medications that could slow down the process and prescribed a drug called Aricept. He also suggested she take a fairly large amount of vitamin E. She sat there smiling as he spoke. My fears were now a reality, and I felt like my world was crumbling down around me. I tried to understand what she must be thinking.

Was she in denial? Did she not comprehend what the doctor was saying? Was she being brave? Did she not believe what he was saying, or was she just rejecting the whole idea? I never was able to answer these questions to my own satisfaction, but after a while, I began to understand that her thought processes were no longer like those of a normal person's. Yes, it was one of the worst days of my life. Whatever the reason, the fact was that she had apparently blocked Alzheimer's out of her mind, and frankly if this was the way she chose to handle it, I saw no benefit in pressing the point.

Later on, when she was feeling confused over some small event, she would ask me in frustration what was wrong with her. I had come to the conclusion, correctly or incorrectly, that *Alzheimer's* was not a word she wanted to hear, and I would hedge my answer with a little bit of nonsense.

"Perhaps the strokes your MRI showed you had suffered are causing a little dementia. What are you worried about? We all get a little confused and forgetful at our age. I'll make a deal with you, you remember the important stuff and I'll take care of the little stuff for both of us, after all we have always been a team, right?"

"I guess," she would answer doubtfully.

"All you really have to remember is what a handsome and intelligent husband you have." She would start to laugh at me because she knew I was kidding her. "If you get too flaky, I'll just put an ad back in the paper for two thirty-two-year-olds."

She would continue to laugh, and I had diverted her away from the feelings of confusion she was having. I have found that humor is a wonderful weapon when dealing with Alzheimer's.

The word *Alzheimer's* was at times inadvertently used in her presence, and she would wear a look of sympathy for the person being discussed, but it was not a word I ever heard her use herself. This type of behavior made me feel there was some kind of awareness going on in her head, but for the most part, she just continued on as though nothing had changed.

She was pleasant as we drove home from the doctor's office. We discussed trivial things, and we even had a few laughs. I attempted to talk about what had just transpired and what the doctor had said, but she ignored me and quickly changed the subject. I didn't know what she was thinking or feeling but I did know, as I said before, that this was definitely not one of the best days of my life.

I filled the prescription for Aricept and bought a good supply of vitamin E as directed. The next day I started giving her the pills, and she offered none of her usual objections to taking medications. I am only guessing, but she must have had some understanding going on in her mind to suddenly have become so cooperative.

I am not sure what I expected the medication to do, but later on I mentioned to the doctor that Terry was still easily confused and forgetful, and I could not detect that it was doing her any good. Her answer was, "But we don't know where she would be without it." I guess that logic made some sense, and I did not blame the doctor, but it was not the most satisfying answer I had ever had given to me.

Actually it seemed to me that in her case the Aricept was causing even more confusion than before. A friend of ours whose husband also suffered from dementia mentioned that she was trying a drug called Exelon and it seemed to be helping. I spoke to Terry's doctor, and we decided to give it a try, but there was no noticeable difference that I could observe. I currently have her on a drug called Reminyl, and this does seem to have slowed down the progression of the disease to some degree.

It should be noted that one drug does not fit all. What works for one patient may not work for another, and experimenting, with the doctor's approval, may be something to consider doing.

It was about October or November of 2003 when I read an article in the newspaper about a drug that had been used in Germany for quite a few years. The article stated that they had had a great deal of success in the treatment of Alzheimer's and had experienced very few side effects. The drug was called Memantine and was not yet available in the United States. It was further stated that the FDA had given the drug its fast go-ahead status, and it was to become available in this country in January of 2004.

I did not want to wait that long, and after surfing the Web on my computer, I located a Canadian pharmacy that carried it, and I placed my order. Surely the drug companies and the FDA must have been aware of this drug considering how long it had been on the market in Germany. Considering its success, I can't help but wonder why it took so long to make it available in this country.

I was thrilled with the immediate improvement I saw in Terry. Prior to taking Memantine, she could not concentrate or focus on a TV program. She would be easily distracted and did not react to the funniest, or saddest, of programs with either laughter or tears. This changed noticeably. She also seemed to recognize family and friends almost immediately, which was something she had been having difficulty with before. Names still gave her a bit of a problem.

This was a fantastic improvement because the TV offered her a source of entertainment that she had lost and could now once again enjoy. Our children were thrilled that their mom could recognize them so quickly and could converse with them a little. It was not a cure, but it did seem to help more than anything else we had tried.

The doctor advised that studies had found that using both Reminyl and Memantine in conjunction with one another seemed to produce the best results. Memantine is now available in the United States under the brand name of Namenda.

I continued to administer Namenda and Reminyl to Terry, but unfortunately after a few weeks, most of its effectiveness gradually diminished, and she slipped back to where she had been before. It was sad to watch it happening, but at least I was able to give her a few more moments of pleasure during the time the drug was effective.

Those of you who have had someone close to you affected by this disease must certainly understand that my primary goal is to do everything in my power to slow down the progress of this terrible affliction. Hope springs eternal, and we strive to buy as much time as possible, praying that a similar drug, or possibly even a cure, is just around the corner.

My Memories Sustain Me

My worst fears had been realized when the doctor told us that it appeared Terry was in the first stages of Alzheimer's. There was an article in the newspaper recently citing a survey that claimed most people feared this debilitating disease more than cancer or heart disease. It was not difficult for me to understand why as I watch my wife's ability to function, both mentally and physically, fade away. If there is any redeeming feature at all in this disease, it is that she no longer seems to be aware of what is happening to her.

I voraciously read everything I can get my hands on that pertains to Alzheimer's, but very little that I read offers much encouragement. There is much discussion about the research in progress to help delay the effects of Alzheimer's. They had developed certain drugs that worked very well on mice but when tested on humans did not work well at all. Unfortunately any mention of a cure was sadly lacking or many years away from being available.

Much of what I read stressed the necessity of caregivers taking care of themselves and resisting any decline into depression. If you do not take care of yourself and you become ill or incapacitated, then you cannot take proper care of your loved one. This was the message they were trying to send, and it made good sense. If something happens to the caregiver, who now takes care of the patient? Admittedly, this advice is much easier said than done.

Terry seemed to tire more easily lately, and she would be grateful when I helped her into her nightgown and tucked her sleepily into bed at about eight o'clock every evening. I had thought that I was getting used to spending my evenings alone after she went to bed, but tonight the loneliness was wearing thin on me. I sat on the couch trying to amuse myself by watching something on TV. It was not a bad show as I recall, but my mind seemed to wander, and I could not really get very interested in the plot.

I guess I was feeling pretty low, and the thought of what Terry had facing her was breaking my heart. I hated watching her deteriorate from the intelligent woman she had once been to the pitiful and lost soul she had become. I felt so sorry for her, and yes, I shamefully admit, for myself also.

As the evening wore on, my eyelids grew heavy, and I dozed fitfully. Inadvertently my mind drifted back to those happier days when Terry and I were first married and we were young and vibrant.

───◈───

After WWII, veterans were returning to civilian life by the thousands and were now marrying the girls they had left behind while they fought the Nazis and Japan. There was an enormous need for affordable housing, and of course, the ensuing demand had caused the price of real estate to skyrocket.

Enter a builder by the name of Alfred Levitt who had a wonderful dream. He envisioned a town made up solely of veterans, their wives, and their children. He built five different and attractive models and did so by applying the Ford method of mass production into building homes. By doing so, he was able to sell homes at prices that were affordable and within the reach of young veterans.

To find land on which he could accomplish this ambition, he looked to the potato farms in a town called Hicksville on Long Island in New York State, and so a bit of GI heaven was born. The homes were well built and landscaped with good sod, shrubs, shade trees, and a variety of fruit trees. The roads were thoughtfully and gracefully curved in order to slow down traffic. This was done for the safety of the many children, he wisely predicted, were certain to come.

Mortgage loans for veterans were available though the government, and the homes sold for the paltry sum of $7990 with mortgage payments of $54 per month. This ridiculously low sum included principal, interest, and taxes. It was here that Terry and I wisely decided to start our married life together and purchased our first home. Eventually these homes rose in price and were selling for close to $250,000.

Our new neighbors were primarily young veterans and their families. They were mostly about our age, and it was not long before new mothers were pushing baby carriages up and down the sidewalks. We too were tempted to start a family, but we cautiously decided to wait a while longer until we could save a bit more money. We also wanted to just enjoy each other for a while and build a better sense of security before bringing a new life into the world.

We waited two years, and then it was here that our first son James Allen (Jimmy or Sep) was born. Our daughter Jil Ann (Jilly or Peanut) soon came along and, last but not least, our youngest son John Louis (Action Jackson).

For some unknown reason that she never explained to me, Terry insisted that all our children's names start with the letter *J*. I could think of no reasonable objection to this, and I liked the names we chose with the letter *J*, so I went along with her wishes.

✦⊰⊱✦

I shifted my body into a more comfortable position and stretched. I could feel some of the loneliness and the stress of my caregiver day slowly seeping away as I recalled these pleasant memories.

Levittown was a great place to raise children, and we became very close to many of our neighbors. We and our children made lifelong friends who became very dear to us. Business and many other reasons eventually caused some of us to move away, but we kept in touch, and distance did not diminish our friendships in any way.

We had barbeques, penny ante card games, and were always ready to give each other a helping hand with any household project. There were no fences in Levittown, and the children would roam from backyard to backyard. The phone would ring, and it would be some neighbor letting us know that the children were all in her backyard playing and were okay. We all extended that courtesy to each other, and no child was ever out of sight of somebody's mother. Tears were wiped away, Band-Aids were distributed freely, and little noses blown indiscriminately by all the mothers.

I stretched again with a large yawn and relaxed a little bit more. A sobering thought entered my mind as I now recalled that some of these wonderful people that had been our close friends and neighbors had passed on. I quickly succeeded in pushing that sad thought from my mind and then suddenly found myself letting out a small chuckle. I remembered the laugh I would get from people when I would kiddingly complain that there was no point in my visiting the old neighborhood anymore. When they would ask me why, I would laughingly explain to them that "all my old buddies are gone, and Terry won't let me visit their widows."

The memories of Levittown slowly passed out of my mind, and my thoughts shifted to the evening I had returned home from the service so many years ago. I think perhaps a tear may have formed in my eye as I recalled the sensation of love and happiness that my parents and I experienced that night.

My mood saddened again as I mourned the fact that they had both passed away at a relatively early age and the only one of their grandchildren they ever really knew was our oldest son Jimmy. They both loved that little boy, and after we would visit with them, my mother would refuse to wash his little fingerprints off the full-length mirror that hung in their entryway. "I feel like he is still here when I see those little fingerprints on the mirror," she would say.

I have always felt badly that my parents and my children never had the opportunity to really know each other. They were gentle and loving people, and I believe that my parents missed something wonderful by not being able to see their grandchildren grow up. My children too never knew the love that would have been bestowed upon them by Mom and Dad.

The only grandparents my children ever really knew were Terry's parents. They too were family prone and loving people. We all enjoyed the company of each other to the extent that eventually the whole family—Terry and I, Grandpa Ray and Grandma Ann, our three children and their spouses, and our seven grandchildren—started to take family vacations together once a year.

I was enjoying my reveries, and I decided to get up and mix myself a highball, something I rarely did and perhaps relax even more. I sat down, took a sip, and allowed my mind to continue remembering some more of the pleasant moments of my life.

Imagine, if you will, an old large but well-kept house on a secluded beach in a small Florida town called Boca Grande. There was a wooden porch with an old love swing built for two on it. I can recall the wonderful moments Terry and I sat there holding hands as we looked out across the clear blue waters of the Gulf of Mexico.

There was something almost magical about that swing. It somehow evoked a wonderful sense of closeness for any couple that quietly sat in it. There was really very little need for conversation at times like this, just being together, relaxed and in love, was all that was required.

There were five bedrooms, four bathrooms, and a large eat-in kitchen. A large picture window in the seashell-decorated rustic living room offering us a beautiful view of the gulf waters as they lapped lazily against the sandy beach. It was a picture that offered a wonderful sense of ease and contentment for us all. Take this beautiful and spacious house, fill it with the people you love most in this world, and you have what all four generations of our family consider a recipe for paradise.

The week that we spent at that house every year allowed the entire family to relax from the rigors of everyday life and simply enjoy each other's company. Grandma Ann and Grandpa Ray loved the place, and the porch swing soon became their favorite spot. They would sit on it like young lovers, and the sweet look of serenity on the faces of those two old people was a lovely sight to behold.

Two of our grandchildren were twins. They were not identical, but it was almost impossible to tell them apart when they were young. When they stood before me, they were to my eye practically carbon copies of each other. I loved to tease them by looking sad and telling them what a shame it was that one of them was so pretty but the other one was so funny looking. They would tease me back by begging me to tell them which one was the funny-looking one. They would point at each other and wink at me when the other twin was not looking as if to say, "She's the funny-looking one, not me."

The whole family got a kick out of them and calling someone in the family "funny looking" became an inside family joke that was actually intended to be more a show of affection than an insult. I would lament the weakness in my nature that caused me to be attracted to funny-looking Italian girls and then look at Terry and shake my head. Everyone would laugh, Terry most of all, and eventually Terry became my funny-looking Italian girl. She loved it.

My heart swelled as I recalled the fun times I had enjoyed with my family in Boca Grande. Those pleasant strolls along the beaches that were sparsely covered with seaweed and looking for pretty seashells. We swam laughingly in the gentle waves as they rolled in, and we fished in the smooth swells of the gulf. In the evening, the men would light up the grill, and we would cook steaks, hot dogs, hamburgers, and if our fishing was successful, we would throw our catches on the grill and feast on delicious fresh fish. The ladies would prepare wonderful side dishes, and we ate like royalty. The highlight meal of the week that we all looked forward to was that one evening during the week when Grandpa Ray would cook up one of his delicious pasta dinners with his great meatballs and Italian sausage.

There was a great deal of good-natured needling and laughter as we enjoyed our meals, and the grandchildren were included in everything we did. All the cousins got along well, and when we were home, they would sleep over at each other's houses periodically. They were comfortable and loved no matter whose home they were in, and it must have seemed to them at times like they all had three sets of parents.

We would clean up after dinner and bring beach chairs down onto the shell-studded shore. The sunsets were spectacular, and we would sit down to watch the sky turn a coral red as the sun sank into the sparkling waters of the gulf. It was a sight that we never seemed to grow tired of and unless it was too cloudy or raining one that we rarely missed.

Grandma and Grandpa are gone now, and we all treasure the golden memories of those days we were able to spend with them. Eventually business and other circumstances made it too difficult for us all to get the same week off every year. The house was too large for just a few of us to rent, and unfortunately the yearly family vacation became an impossibility for us to achieve. We begrudgingly were forced into allowing it to become a pleasure of the past, but the memories linger on.

Terry and I have been fortunate in that we were able to do some traveling before she became ill and been able to take quite a few very fine vacations to some luxurious places, but nothing will ever match the loving closeness we experienced in all those years we vacationed as a family. Yes, we are a close family, and no one has ever had to feel alone. Should an unfortunate circumstance befall any one of us, the whole family is always ready to rally around and offer comfort and support. It has been a difficult time since Terry developed Alzheimer's, and I will be eternally grateful for the sensitivity and support my family has shown me.

I once again stretched my arms over my head, and this time, with a small groan, I opened my eyes wide. I felt revived as I gave thought to all the pleasant memories I had just reviewed. Shame on me, I admonished myself, look at me sitting here felling sorry for myself. Terry and

I have had a wonderful life and been fortunate enough to experience the happiness that only a closely knit family can provide.

There is no denying that fate has presented me and also my family with a very difficult situation. It is a situation in which I am not alone, for many other millions are now in the same boat as I, trying to make their way across the very same stormy sea of despair that I am wallowing in. Life is life, and through no fault of our own, fate will often hand us some seemingly insurmountable heartaches. It is not the heartache that is the real problem. The important problem is how to find the courage that will enable us to handle it.

There have been many bouquets of roses in my life, and a few thorns on the stems were to be expected. It is up to me to determine if I will choose to dwell on the colorful and fragrant beauty of the roses' blossoms, or the painful and ugly wounds the thorns have torn me up with.

Yes, I use my memories to sustain me. They are the life jackets by which I am able to keep my spirits afloat. It is something I know I must do so that I may better care for my funny-looking Italian girl, the loving mother of my children. She is the woman I have loved all my life, but only recently have I really discovered just how much.

Attitudes

They call us caregivers, and we are all part of an army on which fate has played a cruel trick. We are not alone. We number in the many millions, and our numbers are growing every day as the average life expectancy increases. I know that I am not unique, and certainly no saint, but I have concluded that the position I find myself in need not be any harder than I want to make it, or that I will allow it to be.

Life is a precious gift, and we should try to live it to its fullest regardless of what burdens we bare. If we can maintain a good sense of humor and a positive attitude, it is not impossible for us to find pleasure for ourselves and to give pleasure to others. We do what we must the best way we are capable of, and try to do so with a minimum of complaint or self-pity.

Yes, I again admit, this is not an easy thing to do. I live with my wife's Alzheimer's every day, and I am well aware of how difficult this life can be. I only mean to infer that there are some things in life we cannot change, and for our own good and the good of our loved ones, we must find the courage to accept them and go on with life.

Quite often in the course of speaking to other caregivers, many of them will mention how they seem to have developed an odd combination of inner strength and compassion. These are traits that many of us never dreamed we might someday be required to possess. After having heard others speak of these traits, I was surprised to discover that I understood exactly what they were saying. Perhaps you will too.

I have recognized that self-pity is probably the most detrimental attitude that I could adopt for both the well-being of my wife and for myself. I love my wife deeply, and yes, sometimes the pain and anguish I feel for her is almost overwhelming, but I have found that I must do my best not to allow her to see this. I have noticed that she is sensitive to my moods, and if I allow my sadness or any other sign of temperament to show through, she will reflect my moods by also becoming sad and temperamental. Conversely, if I appear happy, she is happy too. Her moods have definitely become a mirror image of my own. It is to both our advantages for me to keep control of my emotions in her presence. I suggest that this is something for everyone to consider. There are moments when my patience wears thin, particularly when I am tired and will snap at her. I feel so guilty when I lose control, but tiredness is part of being a caregiver, and I must accept that I am only human. The best that I can do is to take a deep breath and contritely attempt to make amends.

I have heard others say, "He or she just does that to annoy me." It does seem that way at times, and I too was guilty of this assumption for a short time, but I eventually realized that this was not true. As I mentioned earlier, she does not deliberately do these things because she wants to annoy me. She does them because she is no longer completely rational or in control of her actions.

I have concluded that I am no longer dealing with the mind of an adult that can be reasoned with but more with that of a child who just does not understand. As anyone who has been a parent has probably discovered, patience works better than displaying anger and frustration. If I complain to her about some annoying mistake she has made, all I have succeeded in doing is to make her feel bad and rob her of her dignity. Unlike a child, she is past learning, and the error will soon be repeated no matter what I do or say. This may be one of the most difficult things I have had to learn to accept. I want to see my little girl grow up and be smart again, but I know that barring some miracle this is not to be, and she will revert further and further into infancy.

We have been married many years now, and I used to sometimes tease her that two or three of them have even been good. The truth is that it really has been a good marriage with many wonderful moments. As the doctor said, she did not do anything to cause her illness and is doing her best. I would like to think that something in her mind still knows that I too am doing my best. Fortunately she does not have the ability to be hurt or angry for very long if I slip up. A little gentle humor or teasing can usually bring a smile to her face and all is forgiven and forgotten.

The sulking is gone, and she has become very sweet and docile. Although her eyes often appear blank and unaware, the expression on her face is usually a small pleasant smile, and her entire countenance is one of contentment. I do not know how much she understands, but even so I do not hesitate to tell her that her smile was one of the things about her that I fell in love with. I am well aware that the pleasant personality she had developed with Alzheimer's can often be quite the opposite. I have heard stories of belligerent and difficult behavior that continually grows worse as the disease progresses. I know that I am very fortunate that this has not occurred in our case.

As I watched her illness progress, I tried to self-examine my own personality. I had lived a lifetime in a competitive business environment, which had necessitated my developing a certain amount of firmness. In short, I was not exactly an easy mark. I had faced many a challenge and been able to overcome not all but most of them. My wife's Alzheimer's presented a challenge of a completely different nature than I had ever faced before, and for the first time in my life, I had the sensation of complete helplessness. It was a very humbling experience, and as I looked back, I realized that, with a good deal of effort, I had had to make some very difficult adjustments in my own personality.

I have learned that much of the behavior displayed by Alzheimer's patients depends on which part of the brain is affected. I make no claims that my change of personality and attitude, or my newfound patience and compassion, are the reason for her pleasant disposition, but I cannot help but wonder if they did not, at least, play some small part. People occasionally ask me if she was always as pleasant as she is now, and they are usually surprised when I honestly admit that she was not.

Like most married couples, we did not always agree on how we should raise our children or how our finances should be handled. These were the two main subjects that caused some pretty heated exchanges between us. I can say in all candor that she held up her end of these disputes admirably. She did not hesitate to let me know if she was displeased with something I had done, or said, in no uncertain terms. I too was not shy about stating my views, and we were both fairly strong-willed people. I would angrily tease her by telling her that I knew I had found Mrs. Right when I married her, I just didn't know her first name was Always. The best part of it all was that making up was so much fun. As we matured and our children grew older and more responsible, there seemed to be very few reasons for us to disagree. Money became less of a problem as our earning power increased and the lean years faded behind us. Life was good in those days.

We both always loved to laugh, and a sense of humor was something neither of us was lacking in. Humor has always been one of my staunchest allies in life, and I find that the more often I can find something to make Terry laugh, the more successful my efforts to combat depression and keep both our spirits up are.

I believe that a joke, a pun, or even some gentle teasing requires some degree of thought. It is my intention to try and stimulate her mind in an effort to make her think while she tries to "catch on" to my nonsense. I am sure you have heard it many times before, but I really do believe that laughter is not only the best medicine but also a great medicine. I cannot state with any certainty that what I am doing is any real benefit to her, but it certainly can do her no harm, and we are, at least, having a little fun.

Repetition too seems to breed a sense of familiarity, and when I tell the same old corny jokes to her over and over, she seems to welcome them as old friends that she remembers. I will do whatever it takes to make her happy, and if sometimes I appear to be an idiot in the eyes of others, so be it.

———◆———

There is an excellent book called the *The 36-Hour Day* written by Nancy L Mace, NA, and Peter Rabins, MD, MPH. Much that you will read in my book is no more than an interpretation and application of what I have learned in that book. Although the basics of my methods stem from my own experiences and what I have learned from reading and research, I have also tailored much of what I do to coincide with our own personalities and relationship.

Going On With Life

Although Terry's confusion and memory loss had become fairly obvious, she was still able to function to a reasonable degree. I believed at that time that she could still be trusted not to do anything foolish if I left her alone for the three hours or so it took me to play a short round of golf. She did not seem to mind being left alone for that amount of time, and occasionally I would take her with me just for the ride. We had moved to a golf community where everyone had their own golf cart. It was required that if two people were in the cart, each one must have their own bag. I put a dummy bag on my cart, and she seemed to enjoy the fresh air and just riding along with me. There were times when I would drop an extra ball on the green and try to teach her how to putt. No matter how many strokes she took, she was always thrilled when the ball finally dropped in the hole.

I had read that it was important to try and maintain as much of your usual routines as possible, and so I continued to frequent our favorite restaurants, going to the beach occasionally, and visiting with family and friends. Life was still tolerable. We visited Grandma a couple of times a week at the assisted living facility, and I would often take them out to lunch. Terry had become quite adept at bluffing her way through occasional bad moments and usually behaved pretty well in company if I ran a little interference for her.

It is not unusual for Alzheimer's patients to behave fairly well in a social atmosphere and then revert back to confusion and forgetfulness when they return home. To strangers there sometimes appears to be nothing wrong. I could tell Grandma was still suspicious of Terry's well-being, but to her credit, she no longer made any comments.

Our primary source of enjoyable entertainment stemmed from belonging to a few fraternal organizations. They were convenient meeting places where we were able to socialize with our friends and dance to the music of some of the local bands. These bands played a variety of dance music, most of which was from our era. We had grown up during the war years, and the strains of music from the big band era still lingered in our ears and hearts. We relived those wonderful days of listening to the romantic sounds of bands like Glenn Miller and his "Moonlight Serenade," Harry James playing "It's Been a Long, Long, Time" on his awesomely sweet trumpet, the Dorsey brothers, Benny Goodman, and so many others.

There were crooners like Sinatra, Crosby, and Como along with vocalists like Ella Fitzgerald, Doris Day, and Patti Page. Their diction was perfect, their phrasing was superb, and every word was clearly enunciated. They could tear the heart out of a lonely serviceman who was far from home with songs such as "I'll Be Home for Christmas" and "I Don't Want to Walk Without You."

The teenage girls in those days were called Bobby Soxers. Their style of the day was faded-blue jeans worn with one of their father's white long-sleeve shirts rolled up at the cuffs. Saddle shoes or penny loafers with white socks were considered appropriate wear for the high school girls of this era. What the younger generation calls cool today was called hip back in my day, and dressing this way was considered hip. Each generation makes up its own slang.

The biggest thrill of all was for a group of them to take the train into New York City and go to the Paramount Theater to hear Frank Sinatra croon. They would scream, cry, and swoon as he sang his romantic songs of love to them. He had the fantastic ability of making every girl in the audience feel like he was singing to her and to her alone.

It seemed like only yesterday that we were young, and it was difficult for us to fathom where the time had gone. We were all determined to not allow age to prevent us from enjoying life. We had worked hard all our lives, and we intended to make the most out of our retirement years.

The best way I can describe the fun of belonging to one of these clubs is that it was comparable to going to a wedding reception where there was good food, music, and dancing. There were other members of the clubs that we discovered had been diagnosed with Alzheimer's. Some couples would continue to attend for a short while and then, as the disease progressed, would gradually stop coming because they felt too embarrassed, or distraught, to take their spouses out in public. Others feared they might be imposing on their friends and causing them to feel uncomfortable at the sometimes odd or inappropriate behavior of the Alzheimer's victim. A few tried to keep things as they were before and sit with their old friends while trying to enjoy the evening.

After much consideration, I decided to at least give the latter a try. I reasoned that in the event our friends displayed any signs of embarrassment or discomfort at all I could always bow out gracefully and leave. I sought to avoid change as much as possible. I did not want to give up on living life for Terry or myself any sooner than was absolutely necessary. I intended to continue doing the things we both had both enjoyed doing for as long as possible.

It was impossible for our friends not to have noticed over time that Terry's personality had changed. Of course they were deeply distressed when I took them aside and quietly informed them of Terry's diagnosis, but it obviously came as no great surprise to them. Most of them had suspected something was wrong for quite some time. We had been active members and were pretty well known by many of the members of the various clubs we belonged to. Bad news travels fast, and it did not take long for word about Terry to get around. I worried about the reaction of my fellow members and despised the thought of any pitiful glance that might furtively come our way.

Terry had lost the ability to do many everyday things without assistance. I found I had to assist her in choosing what she should wear for an evening out and then help her to dress. I tried hard to remember the combinations of clothing she liked best in order to keep her appearance as attractive as it had always been. I had seen how some Alzheimer's victims had been allowed to let their appearance deteriorate, and I was determined that I would not let this happen to Terry.

Terry had always enjoyed dancing, and I had learned to enjoy it too. Although Fred Astaire and Ginger Rogers would never lose any sleep for fear we would replace them on the stage, we did manage to become quite passable on the dance floor. It was a dancing crowd, and some of the members would occasionally bring their visiting sons or daughters from up north to the clubs for an evening of fun. The young visitors would be amazed to see people in their seventies, eighties, and even in their nineties get up to dance the fox trot, waltz, or sway their hips to the many Latin rhythms such as the rumba, cha-cha, or perhaps even a tango.

I believe that these older people are not just dancing because they happen to be in good shape for their age. They are in good shape because they go dancing and probably have been dancing all their lives. Staying active is one of the main reasons these senior citizens are still going strong and enjoying life.

I am aware that many men consider dancing to be something less than masculine, and I could not disagree more. I have played sports such as golf, tennis, bowling, and many other athletic endeavors. I place dancing as a sport that requires the same coordination, stamina, and imagination as any other sport. Consider this. Dancing is the only sport in which you have the added enjoyment of holding an attractive female in your arms. Seems pretty masculine to me.

In addition to being good physical exercise, it is also a good mental exercise as you try to remember or learn new steps. The thing about dancing that I liked the most was that it seemed to please Terry. She would brighten up noticeably at the sound of the music and laughter. I believe it was therapeutic for her and kept her going to some degree.

Terry had always been a very private and conservative person, and although she was lovable at home, she had always avoided any public display of affection. Alzheimer's seemed to have subdued many of her inhibitions. For example, if the band played a romantic melody while we were dancing, she would now surprise me by tilting her head up wanting to steal a little kiss. The first time this happened, I glanced around to see if anyone had noticed. I was pleased when I discovered that yes, we had been caught in the act, but those who had caught our little display of affection were nodding and smiling with approval.

Terry was also at the point where she needed some assistance in eating. When our food was served, I would cut up her meat for her; then I would put a fork in her hand and let her try to eat by herself while I ate some of my food. It was difficult for her, and after a few bites, she would give up. I would then gently take the fork away from her and feed her myself. Everyone at the table pretended not to notice, and she was not aware enough to be embarrassed.

After a few dances, we would sit down and rest. Sometimes I would notice that something was bothering her. I knew her well and how quickly her mind could play tricks on her. She could go from happy and fairly lucid to confused and frightened in a heartbeat.

I asked her if anything was wrong. It only took at moment for me to realize she had lost what little memory she still had for the moment when she asked me my name and then confided in me that she was not sure she had a place to stay that night. She had gone from knowing me well enough to show me affection on the dance floor to wondering who I was and where she lived. Still, she must have felt some connection in order to trust me enough to ask those questions.

"Why, honey," I tried to soothe her, "we have been married for many years, and I am your husband, Lou. We have a nice home where we live with our mottled cat Fernando. You know I love you, and you have nothing to worry about because I will always take good care of you. Come on now, stop being silly and let's have another dance."

I think it may have been the mention of our cat that stirred her memory and eased her concern.

"Oh, thank God, I guess I forgot," she answered.

On the way home, she did not seem to recognize any of the familiar landmarks we were passing and had passed before after many years of traveling the same roads.

"Are you sure you know where you are going?" she asked.

Most of the time, probably because she knows me so well, she still has the ability to know when I am teasing her, and I can usually draw a laugh out of her.

"Oh my gosh," I answered, "I thought you knew the way home. I guess we are lost."

"Stop it now," she would say half fearfully, but she saw me smiling and she too had a laugh in her voice.

About this time we were pulling into our garage.

"I don't know how you do it," she said in amazement, "you always seem to find the way home."

How strange this disease is, how does she even remember I always find the way home?

"It was the automatic homing device in the car," I told her.

"You're crazy," she answered.

"I know, aren't you glad?"

She answered with a little giggle, "Yes, I am."

Perhaps this kind of behavior may sound foolish to some, but I do it to make her laugh and give her a moment of pleasure. I am hopefully making her use her mind with my teasing and nonsense. I admit, I have no way of knowing if it is of any help or use, actually I doubt that it is, but I cannot help myself from at least trying to exercise her brain. Perhaps it will keep her with me a little longer.

We continue to go dancing and to socialize with our friends. Any skepticism I may have had as to what their reaction might be was soon proven to be unfounded. Our friends, nodding acquaintances, and even perceptive strangers were wonderfully compassionate and caring. It was rare evening that at least a few people did not come over to the table where we were sitting with our friends. They would take time from their dancing to say hello, ask how we were doing, and often give Terry a small hug that was sometimes accompanied by a little kiss on the cheek.

Should Terry have a need to visit the ladies' room, a few of the other ladies would also suddenly decide they had the same urge and accompany her. They knew I could not take her and that she probably would not be able to find her way back to the table or possibly not even be able to find a stall.

I cannot say enough good things about these wonderful people who proved themselves to be our true friends with their actions. Their understanding and sincere concern made what could have been an embarrassing and difficult situation something that enabled Terry, and myself, to be able to continue socializing. My faith in human nature has increased a hundred fold since Terry has fallen prey to Alzheimer's. I never imagined there were so many good people in this world who were ready and willing to pass out a "cough drop" to a friend in need.

Yes, they were wonderful friends, but there were times when I felt guilty that perhaps I was imposing on them. I wondered if my desire to keep things as they were was not causing me to unwittingly take advantage of them.

I decided to at least cut back on our evenings out and possibly eventually stop completely. One evening I mentioned to our friends that I thought perhaps going out every week was too much for Terry and I was thinking of cutting back. "Don't worry if we don't show up next week," I said.

They knew me pretty well and suspiciously asked why I had come to this conclusion. "She seems to have a good time when she is with us, and if she tires, you always take her home. What makes you think it's too much for her?"

When I did not answer because I did not know what to say, they continued.

One of the women saw through me and spoke up, "If you are wanting to do this because you think we mind helping out, forget it. Terry needs this evening out, and so do you. Don't you know we all love Terry?"

Everyone nodded their heads in agreement, and one of the men let out a loud groan. "We may all love Terry, but you I'm not too sure of, Lou." Everyone started to laugh.

"Come to think of it, I guess we would all suffer from withdrawal if we didn't have your corny jokes to listen to."

Now everyone was really laughing at me. He had taken the edge off the moment by simply breaking my chops. Yes, I laughed, but there were tears of happiness in my eyes.

Robert Browning wrote, "Come grow old with me! The best is yet to be. Youth is but the half."

No Man Is An Island

When we first moved to Florida, we rented an apartment for about nine months to make certain we liked living here. We checked out the various lifestyles and eventually found a lovely condo right on the shores of Tampa Bay. The view of the water was breathtaking, and we enjoyed the casual carefree life that condo living afforded us.

Our bedroom faced the east, and when we awoke in the morning, we could see the sunrise painting the skies with delicate hues of beautiful pastel colors. Many mornings we could look out over Tampa Bay and see dolphins gracefully swimming by as they surfaced for air.

Sometimes, after a rainstorm, something I had never witnessed before would occur. Double rainbows would form, and separating them would be a band of pitch-black sky. Their beauty was breathtaking. Tampa has been called the lightning capital of the world, and a thunderstorm at night across the bay and over the city was an electric display of flashing light that no man could possibly duplicate. In the winter, when the tide was low, there would be a colorful array of water fowl on the beach—white egrets, seagulls, pink-colored roseate spoonbills, and blue herons mixed in with the seagulls.

We loved our little corner of what we considered to be paradise, and we were quite content there for quite a few years until Terry's condition noticeably started to slowly decline. Recently she seemed to be having some difficulty in keeping her balance, and she would extend her arms out to steady herself. On one occasion I saw her pause and appear to be teetering at the top of the staircase leading down from our second-story condo.

This concerned me greatly. I hated the thought of leaving our comfortable little condo that we loved so much, but with a good deal of agonizing, I realized that Terry's safety had to come first. I considered selling our second-story condo and trying to find one for sale on the ground floor in order to stay in the complex. I soon discarded this idea because the many mangrove trees along the shore blocked the view of the water from the ground floor, and it just was not the same.

With the realization that Terry's condition was worsening, an added consideration came into play. Our three children all lived fairly close to each other in a town called Palm Harbor, which was about thirty minutes north of us. It really was not all that far, but in the event of an emergency, I felt time might be of the essence, and I wanted them to be able to reach us quickly.

We started to hunt for another place closer to them that would suit our specific needs. I found a nice little two-bedroom, two-bath house with a two-car garage. I wanted a small place because Terry's ability to keep house was rapidly waning, and I knew that eventually all the work would fall on me. Housekeeping was not one of my favorite sports.

The house was located on a cul-de-sac, which offered very little traffic in case Terry began to wander. It was not something she had started to do yet, but I had heard many stories of patients wandering at the support group meetings, and I knew that wandering and getting lost was not unusual for people in her condition. I decided that I would not take the chance on her starting to wander, and this place seemed to be relatively safe. Everything that I needed in a home was there. I felt my purpose had been served because now all my children's homes were within easy reach of us.

In the beginning, when we first moved into our new home, Terry was still capable of functioning pretty well. The Alzheimer's seemed to be progressing very slowly, probably because at this stage the medication she was taking did seem to be helping, and she was usually fairly aware of what was going on around her. The process was so slow that it was hardly noticeable, and it was difficult for me realize that she was slowly becoming a little more unsure of herself and a little more dependent on me. I was hardly aware that I was having to give her more assistance today with something that she had been capable of doing, without too much trouble, yesterday.

Our daughter suggested that we install an emergency alarm system where we had only to press a red button to get help. It was a good idea because of the possibility of my getting another heart attack, although my checkups were fine, was something to consider. If something happened to me, then Terry would be left alone and in her state might not be able to help herself or me.

We hoped that by not having to use the phone, which she had difficulty with, and possibly just having to press a button might be something she could handle. We practiced it with her, and she seemed capable of performing this simple task. The system also came with a pendant that could be worn around the neck. This pendant also had a red button that would alert the emergency service if we needed help.

We became friendly with our next-door neighbors and discovered they had a problem similar to ours. Our problem was, of course, Alzheimer's, and their problem was that the gentleman next door had suffered from a stroke. His symptoms were very similar to Alzheimer's. He was confused in his thinking, he had difficulty completing a sentence, and he too had difficulty with his balance. They were good people, and with both of us having these similar problems, we quickly became good friends.

The community we chose to move into had three nine-hole, par thirty executive golf courses. They were well kept and sufficiently challenging for even low handicap golfers. A round of golf could usually be accomplished in a short three hours, and it was perfect for someone in my situation.

As I mentioned earlier, Terry was still functioning well enough to not get herself in any trouble, and at that time I believed she was mentally capable of being left alone for the three hours it took me to complete a round of golf. Fortunately nothing went wrong, but I know now that it was a mistake and not at all a wise thing for me to do considering how quickly they can become confused.

I did not continue to do this for very long as I realized her confusion was actually continuing to worsen, and I became increasingly worried and uneasy about my leaving her alone, even for a short time. Reluctantly I decided to give up my golf until I could make proper arrangements for someone to stay with her while I was gone. I interviewed a few women but did not find anyone that I felt really comfortable with. My neighbor noticed that I was not playing golf anymore and asked me why. I answered truthfully that I was concerned about leaving Terry alone and informed her that I was investigating the possibility of hiring someone to stay with her so I could get away for a few hours.

She surprised me when she immediately volunteered to sit with Terry while I golfed. I thanked her for being so thoughtful but told her I felt it would be too much of an imposition on her. She refused to take no for answer and insisted that she would enjoy having Terry's company in the morning. I began to weaken.

She continued to persist. "My husband is a late riser, and he rarely wakens until about 11:00 a.m.," she stated. "On the other hand, I am an early riser and usually rise about 6:00 a.m. every morning. I know you try to get early tee times and are usually home by eleven thirty," she urged.

It would be no problem for her, she insisted, and she would love to have Terry for company while her husband slept. I was skeptical, but I had to admit that the timing was perfect for both of us. I continued to resist for fear that I would be taking advantage of her, but she was adamant and finally persuaded me into at least giving it a try.

I started to bring Terry next door on my two golf days. I would bring her over shortly after 7:00 a.m. I would have her all dressed and fed by then. My neighbor's husband was alert enough to be trusted not to do anything foolish if he should awake while she was gone, and she had no problem leaving him alone if she wanted to go out with Terry. The two ladies would watch T.V. for a while, and then when the stores opened, they would go out for a pleasant stroll through the mall and window-shop. The highlight of their morning was taking a leisurely break for coffee and a doughnut. They are home and waiting for me by the time I finish playing golf and anxious to tell me about the bargains they saw on their little outing.

I look at them skeptically.

"Yeah sure," I said, "Two good-looking chicks like you just out innocently window-shopping, Ha! A likely story, I bet you're out eyeing and flirting with all the men and looking for a little action."

They protest and shriek with laughter. They know I am teasing them. "You're nuts," they say. I get a kick out of hearing them laugh and watching them roll their eyes while they deny my accusations.

My neighbor was doing me a tremendous favor, and I knew it, but any attempt to compensate her financially would have been considered an insult. I tried to find ways to reciprocate by helping her out with household chores that her husband could no longer perform. I had always been pretty handy, and I was happy to perform simple tasks such as cleaning up fallen branches in her yard after a storm, opening a jar, climbing a ladder to replace a lightbulb, and on one occasion replacing the valves in her toilet tank.

We all go out to dinner together quite often, and we will usually have a cocktail before dinner. Her husband enjoys it when I call him my favorite drinking buddy and we clink glasses.

She has back problems, and there are times when she must undergo certain procedures at her doctor's office and is not allowed to drive afterward. Once again I am glad to help and drive them there and back. As you can see, I do what I can, but I know I can never fully repay her for the help she gives me with Terry. I know now that no matter how much I loved my wife, I needed the relief my neighbor gave me from the stress of constantly caring for Terry. I also know that I am now capable of finding more patience and I am doing a better job of caring for her by being able to get some relief and pursuing some of my own interests.

If we are fortunate enough to have reached a certain point in life, the reality of aging is something we will eventually have to face. Terry was the one who was ill now, but as I mentioned, for her sake, I had to consider the possibility of my becoming ill, perhaps being hospitalized, or even passing away. What would happen to Terry if I was no longer able to care for her?

I started to investigate my various options. Fate had already thrown us a curve ball, and I wanted to prepare for whatever it had in store for us in the future. I know my children would have stepped in if some catastrophe should befall me, but I did not want to place them in the difficult position of making decisions I should have taken care of in advance. I regret now that I had not been more aware of long-term health insurance. The assisted living facilities were good, but most of them required that the patient be reasonably able to care for themselves. Although Medicaid did have a plan to financially assist in the cost, it was difficult to come by, and the amount offered was not very sufficient.

I was shocked when I discovered that the average cost for placing the patient in a nursing home could run anywhere from $50,000 to as high as $80,000 per year at that time. A sum that would be virtually impossible for many, if not most, people. Medicaid could assist financially, but your eligibility depended primarily on the amount of your assets and income. (I learned later on that the use of an elder law attorney was useful if not absolutely necessary to qualify—more about this later.)

Although some of the facilities seemed quite attractive and adequate, many of the ones I inspected seemed to be badly understaffed, which in turn does not speak well for patient care. I also looked into various agencies that offered day care in the home and found that the average charge ranged from about $15 to $17 per hour and even more for nights. Another option was to hire a live-in to help assist in the care of the patient along with some cooking and housework. This, I realized, entails a loss of privacy, and I was not particularly comfortable with it.

My neighbor continues to help, and in addition I started using an agency one day a week for seven hours to see how Terry would react. In a way, it was a test. They send the same woman every week, and she seemed to have developed a sincere affection for Terry. As I mentioned, Terry is quite docile and not difficult to handle. She too, just as my neighbor does, enjoys taking Terry to the mall and sometimes to the beach for walks, and then they have lunch together. Part of the service is a little housekeeping, and she cleans my kitchen, does the dishes, the bathroom tile floors, and the vacuuming. She is good humored and keeps Terry laughing and happy.

I have attempted to ease my situation as much as possible, and I do believe that by doing so I have been able to keep the hidden negative emotions I spoke of earlier in check. I have found the ability to put on a cheerful countenance in Terry's presence and to keep her content and well cared for. I often wonder if I would have been able to maintain this facade if I had not heeded the wise advise of others and found a little time for myself.

Support groups are also an excellent form of therapy for the caregiver. I found a facility that met on the second Tuesday of the month at 3:30 p.m. They had wisely set up a system of keeping the patients entertained so that the caregivers could attend the meeting. I worried that I might upset Terry if I told her what the meeting was really about, and although I had always tried to be honest with her, I had learned that, for her sake, it was sometimes better to tell a little white lie. I had told Terry that I had to attend a business meeting and that I was bringing her along so she could enjoy herself chatting with some of the other wives while I was busy. With tongue in cheek, I called it therapeutic fibbing.

I had called in advance to say I was coming, and on the second Tuesday of that month, I drove over to the facility. A pleasant-looking woman approached me, and I introduced myself. She welcomed me and then turned to Terry and gave her a big smile while she started to chat with her. In a few moments, she took Terry by the hand, and to my relief, Terry had no objections as they marched happily off together.

I entered the room I was directed to and found an empty seat at a large oblong table at which about ten people were seated. An attractive woman sat at the head of the table who was obviously the facilitator. She introduced herself and informed us of her various credentials. She asked us each to introduce ourselves, say who it was we were taking care of, and to please explain what we had done for ourselves this week.

I was pleased with that request: "What had we done for ourselves this week?" It struck me that it seemed to give credence to my own philosophy of caregivers taking better care of themselves in order to take better care of their loved ones. It eased some of my guilt I sometimes felt about leaving her with my neighbors and the agency woman.

There were three other men at the table besides myself. The rest were women. All of the men and a few of the women had permanently placed their charges in the facility we were at for the meeting. They all felt they had made the right decision as they told their stories and spoke of the difficulty and guilt they experienced in letting go. One man confided that after the first three weeks he felt so guilty that he was about to take his wife back home again. He was grateful now that friends and family had talked him out of it. He was satisfied now that she had adjusted well and was being well taken care of. He admitted that with the entertainment programs the facility offered, perhaps they were doing a better job than he had been able to do himself.

"The day I made the decision to place her here was the worst day of my life," he said, "but it was the right one.

A young woman whose mother suffered from Alzheimer's tearfully exclaimed how she hated the disease that was making her mother so difficult to handle, and robbing her of her dignity and independence.

I wondered if perhaps it might not be even more difficult for a younger person, such as she, to face the inevitability of some illness and possibly even death befalling a parent they have loved and respected for so long.

"What a horrible disease," she painfully exclaimed.

Those who had placed their loved ones in the facility had done so for various reasons. Some were in poor health themselves and lacked the strength and physical ability to lift their loved ones if required. Most agreed that they had probably kept their loved ones home longer than they should have. They had all agonized and suffered pangs of guilt when the heartbreaking time finally came and the hard decision could no longer be put off. They felt that they were doing what was best, not only for themselves, but also what was best for their loved ones.

Except for an occasional comment, the facilitator offered little in the way of advice, preferring to let everyone have their say. Experiences were compared, and in many cases, the characteristics of the problems were similar enough for someone else to relate how they had handled the same problem. I was able to absorb quite a bit of useful information and continued to come once a month. They were primarily a group of people who were experiencing the same stressful emotions and trying to give support and aid to each other.

It is not a "misery loves company" meeting, nor are these people looking for sympathy. It is simply a demonstration of human nature at its best, people with similar problems showing compassion and love for their fellowman.

For those who had succumbed and placed their spouses full-time in the facility, the loneliness they were experiencing at their loss seemed to be a big problem. After years of married life, things had changed drastically for them. The companionship and the intimacy they had once known was now a thing of the past, and it was very depressing for them. Friends would occasionally invite them along to dinner or a party, but most felt like a fifth wheel, missing their mate and feeling more alone than ever.

One woman whose husband had been in a nursing home for quite a few years hesitantly admitted that she was beginning to consider the possibility of dating for companionship. Men friends had asked her out, but so far, her conscience had caused her to decline their invitations.

"I am not getting any younger, and I hate the idea of spending the rest of my life alone," she said, "I still love my husband deeply, but would it be such a terrible thing if I allowed a male friend to take me out to dinner?"

One of the men cleared his throat and spoke up, "I know exactly how she feels. I too love my wife, and I visit her almost every day to see that she is comfortable and being well taken care of. The truth is that most of the time she is not aware of who I am or that I am even present. If I were to find a lady friend who understood my loneliness, or perhaps even was experiencing something similar herself, would it be so wrong if I allowed myself to enjoy her company for an evening, to have a little conversation and perhaps a few laughs. I would be taking nothing away from my wife. She is no longer aware of anything I do. I too am growing older. Do I not have the right to try and find some enjoyment and happiness in my few remaining years?"

There was silence in the room for a moment. It was obvious that there were many mixed emotions. A few people nodded their heads and admitted they had experienced the same thoughts. A few others sat in silent disagreement with very serious faces. I realized that I had not yet walked in his shoes, and I tried not to be judgmental, but I did not believe it was something I could ever do.

Terry was not as far along as many of the others. She still knew me and was able to converse with me. She was still some company to me and could laugh at my jokes and understand much of what I might say to her. I listened with interest to what the others were saying, but I had not as yet looked that far into the future. Now I began to wonder how I would handle it if the day came when I had to place Terry in a facility. The realization of how terrible the loneliness must be for these people really penetrated my mind for the first time. Was this then what I had to look forward to? I could not imagine a life without Terry in it. I did not sleep well that night.

Our Family

Time has passed, and Terry has reached the stage where she is no longer sure of who I am, who her children are, or who her friends are. It is a strange affliction because even though she does not know who we are, she is always pleased to see us. We feel there must be some connection left in her that causes a semblance of recognition. She continues to ask me where her husband is and is skeptical when I tell her I am her husband. I will try to convince her of who I am by telling stories about things we have done together, how many years we have been married, how many children we have, and how well I knew her parents and other relatives. I try to stir her memory by reminding her of cute little happenings in our children's lives. She often gives me a perplexed look.

"How do you know all that? Is it really you?" she might say as she looks me over. We all try hard to overlook and accept her forgetfulness and confusion. What else can we do?

I see my three children bravely attempt to force a smile as they try to suppress their feelings. Try as they might, they cannot hide the hurt in their eyes as a terrible realization confronts them. Their once loving and intelligent mother no longer recognizes them or even knows their names. They too will use the same tactics that I do by trying to remind her of some of the little antics they performed when they were young. They too can sometimes get a small reaction.

She seems to be happiest when we are all together. Her eyes brighten, and she wears an almost constant smile. She laughs at the joking around we do whether she understands what is going on or not, and when we laugh, she laughs.

Occasionally she will become a little frustrated and ask, "What's wrong with me? Sometimes I feel so dumb."

When this happens, my only explanation is that she is just having an occasional lucid moment. Something must click in her mind, and a certain awareness probably enters her mind that tells her all is not well.

It is always momentary, but at times like these, I cannot help but feel a strong wave of affectionate compassion course through me. I feel so badly for her, and I hurt to the depths of my soul. She is missing out on so much, and I feel so sorry for her as I remember the woman she once was.

"It is just the small strokes the doctor said you experienced that have caused you to be a little slower than you used to be. I'm not that fast myself anymore," I tell her, and I try to ease her out of it. "It really doesn't matter because you are still beautiful, and we all love you."

She smiles at me, but I can see her eyes slowly growing bland again, and I know that she is drifting back to her lost state. Actually it is rare that she shows any real signs of awareness that anything is really wrong with her.

Watching the mind of someone you love disintegrate is a heartbreaking experience for the whole family. We try to insulate ourselves from the pain, each in his or her own way. We hide our feelings from each other attempting not to cause any additional pain to the others while we each go through our own private hell. We cannot run away from our feelings because they follow us no matter how far we flee. We simply strive to find the courage to face them and learn to live with them.

Someone at the last support group meeting asked if suppressing our feelings from our families was a wise thing to do. Was it good to do this, or was it better to perhaps relieve some of our emotions by letting our true feelings come out and giving them the opportunity to express theirs? It was an interesting question. There was quite a discussion among us, but unfortunately no really acceptable conclusion surfaced. Was suppressing our true feelings to each other really the path to pursue? Would letting a little steam off possibly offer a safety valve to alleviate some of the inner pressure we all were feeling?

One evening after we and our family had gotten together for a potluck dinner, we retired to the family room to watch a little TV and chat a little. Terry had eaten well, and it was not long before she started to nod and finally dozed off. Her appetite had been diminishing lately, and we were all pleased that she had eaten well tonight. It was not unusual for her to doze off like this, and I think we were all happy to see her relaxed and comfortable. My oldest son Jim commented that she had sure eaten well tonight.

"Yeah! It was the dish that I brought that she liked best though," my daughter Jil kidded.

"Sure it was, I knew you were going to say that," Jim answered back in annoyance, and we all laughed.

Typical brother and sister banter.

"How are you doing, Dad?" Jack asked.

The question of suppressing our feelings that had been asked at the meeting came to my mind, and I decided to do a little testing. I paused for a moment before answering.

"I'm doing okay, I guess. To tell the truth I have been doing a little soul-searching and trying to fathom what I am really feeling. If there is one thing in life that I feel I have some right to be proud of, it is you, my family. You have all been wonderful and supportive of Mom and I, and I cannot thank you enough for that. Just your being here and visiting makes life easier for me.

"The truth is that when I see Mom like this, it hurts like crazy, and I know it hurts you too. I can see the hurt in your eyes as you watch your mom fade away, and it is one of the things that trouble me the most. We bravely try not to show our feelings to each other, and perhaps that is as it should be, perhaps I should not be talking to you this way, but I thought that maybe, just this once, it might help to relieve some of the pressure I feel and have tried to keep subdued and hidden by letting off a little steam and saying some things that you probably all already know anyway.

"I think it is only natural that Mom meant something different to all of us, and we all have our own private memories of her. She is my wife, and I guess I just want to hear myself say out loud how much I miss the woman that once was my trusted companion, my best friend, and my lover.

"We lived together day in and day out for many years. We enjoyed the many good times we had together and faced the bad times that inevitably must fall into the lives of everyone. We laughed together, and we cried together. We were joined as one, and now I am left with a terrible void that I know will only worsen. It is a void that our compassionate friends can only try to understand, but it is one of those things in life that must actually be experienced to be really understood."

I paused and looked at the faces of my sons and daughter. I could see I had their full attention.

"To each of you she was your mom, and your relationship with her was not the same as mine. You have moved on, and you all now have your own families and are making your own memories. I have opened up much of what I am feeling to you, partially to see if there was something you too would like to get off your chest, and partially to see if it might not somehow offer me some relief and make me feel better."

There was dead silence for a moment. I could see that they were all taken aback by my little recitation. I was usually pretty upbeat, and they were not used to hearing me talk this way. I wondered if I had made an error in judgment. Perhaps I just should have stayed quiet.

"And has it made you feel better dad?" one of them finally asked.

I hesitated with my answer for a moment while I gave it some thought.

"You know, oddly enough, I think it did. I do feel somewhat relieved. I guess I have not said anything to you that you had not already known, but saying it out loud has helped to some degree."

Once again the room grew silent as each of us became lost in our own thoughts.

It was Jim our oldest son who first broke the silence. I think it was a surprise to all of us because Jim was usually quite reticent. He cleared his throat, and with his head slightly bowed, he began to speak softly to us. He did not want to wake Terry.

"Of course you're right, Dad, we are all hurting for Mom, but I don't think it's not only because we are protecting each other but also because it is so hard to put into words what we are really feeling.

"When I think of Mom now, I cannot help but see her as she is now. It is not the image of her that I want to see or remember her by. I find myself wanting to push that picture out of my mind. I want to remember her as she used to be, full of life, smart, and loving. I hate it that she often no longer knows who I am. I know she cannot help it, but it troubles me greatly. It does not seem possible that my own mom does not know me. My loving mom who thought I could do no wrong. The mom who always pleaded my defense when you, Dad, got angry with me because I had not done well on a report card or misbehaved in some other way."

He stopped for a moment and swallowed hard before he continued.

"My mouth waters when I think of the delicious meals she cooked every night and how she could bake the best apple pie I ever tasted. I still remember the love that was in her heart for us and her grandchildren. She was always happy to take care of our children if my wife Dianne and I wanted to get away for a few days. She never said no, and it was great for us to be able to take a little vacation by ourselves.

"Now that I am older and have children of my own, I can understand the sacrifices you both made. The things you denied yourselves during the lean years so that you could give more and do more for us, your children. I'm a grown man now, old enough to have experienced a few bumps in life myself, but I do miss the mom I once knew. I feel so helpless and frustrated that there is nothing I can do to help her overcome her illness. There are few things in life that I can think of that ever hurt me more than seeing her this way."

Once again he lowered his eyes as we all sat quietly. Yes, as I said, Jim was not usually given to talking so openly, preferring to keep his thoughts mostly to himself, and I think we were all a bit surprised at what he had said. All of our hearts were aching for him, and for ourselves, as we pondered all that he had so lovingly and sincerely expressed.

We all turned to Jack, our youngest, as he suddenly started to speak.

"I know what you mean, Jim. It's almost like she is gone already. It is hard to believe the woman we see now is the same woman who did all those wonderful things for us. I think of those things a lot lately. I know it sounds silly, but oddly enough, the one thing that constantly creeps into my mind is how she was never too busy to stop whatever she was doing and make her always hungry teenager a sandwich. I can't remember her ever saying, 'Make it yourself.' I sometimes think maybe she should have. Crazy how the little things come to mind.

"I think of the times when my wife Patti or I would receive a call from our children's school informing us that one of our girls was feeling ill. We would phone Mom and Dad and ask them to please pick up their ailing grandchild from class. They would take her to their home for Mom to lovingly nurse until we finished working at our jobs and could come and pick her up."

Jack looked at me and said, "You and Mom were always there for us no matter what, and you have made more than one dream come true for us. I was deeply troubled for a while because I no longer knew how to show my love for her. She does not remember that I am her son, and I feared I would frighten her if I dared to take her in my arms and give her a hug. Imagine being afraid to show affection for your own mother. I asked Dad what he thought about this, and he told me he felt that there was still enough of a connection that a little hug would not frighten her, and he was right. I have so many good memories of her, and I too miss the mom I once knew."

Our daughter Jil had listened closely, nodding occasionally as her brothers spoke. I had watched her face and could only surmise what she must have been feeling.

I had very mixed feelings about the wisdom of my having started this, but it was too late to stop things now. Each word that that the boys had uttered must have been like another turn in the valve that was slowly opening the floodgates of Jil's emotions.

She started slowly, but the words that she had evidently been holding in for so long could no longer be denied, and suddenly they came gushing forth in a quiet and deeply sincere manner that drew our complete attention.

"I feel a slow grieving process as I see myself losing my mom little by little. I see the confused look in her eyes, and I try to console myself with the thought that at least she is still here with us and she is still my mom.

"I suppose it is a form of denial because the reality is that although she is still here in body, the person I could always trust and go to for motherly advice is gone. I can no longer tell her my problems or phone her to help me remember one of her great recipes. Most of all, I miss the unconditional love she always supplied me with as only a mother can. I would love to be able to carry on an intelligent conversation with her again and talk about past memories. We were so close, and now she can no longer remember her little girl, her teenager, or her adult daughter who now has a family of her own. I went from daughter to best friend to no one. Yet I know there is some recognition because she is always glad to see me and is comfortable with me as we attempt to converse.

"'I haven't seen you in such a long time,' she will say, but it is only a reflex conversation because I may have seen her only the day before. When I leave her, she will welcome a hug and a kiss from me. 'I hope you come back for a visit soon,' she will say."

Jil paused for a moment while she struggled with her emotions. Her brothers and I sat quietly as she so eloquently expressed many of our own feelings better than we could ourselves. We could feel the passion in her words as she spoke, her voice sometimes cracking and her eyes glistening with moisture.

"I feel so badly that Mom has lost so much by not being able to watch her grandchildren grow up. They all loved Nana as she loved them, but they knew her for such a short time while they were young. This horrible disease has prevented them from really knowing her and the woman she was as she slowly faded away. What pride she would have taken in all of their achievements, how happy she would have been to shower them with love and perhaps spoil them a little. She was a wonderful grandmother before she became ill, and it is not only her loss but that of the grandchildren too. Communication is so difficult, and she has difficulty completing a sentence. Her ability to enjoy life has lessened no matter how hard we try to entertain her. She can no longer enjoy a day at the beach or have the pleasure of cooking dinner for her family, which was something she once loved to do. She has lost the productivity she once prided herself in.

"Mom took such good care of herself. She ate right and watched her weight. She exercised, played a good game of tennis, and enjoyed dancing. She led a good, healthy life, and I cannot understand why something like this would happen to someone like her. I remember how proud I was of her when she attained an AA degree in accounting, working during the day and going to college in the evening at the age of fifty. She was still all right then, but unfortunately Alzheimer's has no respect for intelligence. To have gone from the bright woman she was then to what she is today is almost unbelievable and close to being unbearable. I think of the mom who cared for my oldest child Justin while I was in the hospital having my premature twin daughters. After they were born, she came over every Tuesday night after work to help me with them so I could get some rest."

Jil paused and looked directly at me.

"I am sad for you too, Dad. You have shown your love for us in many ways, and now you are proving your love for your wife. I think we all admire your transformation from the man who was once taken care of by his wife to the role of the caregiver who now takes care of her every need. We know you do your best to stay cheerful and try to keep Mom and us laughing. The fact that you have told us of your true feelings tonight was very unlike you and I think took us all by surprise. We probably all realized how you felt, but to have it voiced out loud by you came as a complete surprise. I think we all realize the strain this must be putting on you, and we worry about your health too. Although you seem to have recovered from your heart attack, we are concerned with the constant stress we know you are under. We admire how you have been smart enough to do as your doctor says in order to take care of Mom. You too watch your diet, exercise, and try to keep both you and Mom active socially. You better keep it up because we don't want to lose you too. I'm watching you."

I was pleased to see a little smile break out on her face as she said "I'm watching you."

Terry was beginning to stir, and we all glanced over at her, causing Jil to stop talking. The boys had allowed some of what they were feeling to be exposed, but it seemed to me that it was Jil who had given the situation the most thought. I had not realized how much everyone had been carrying around. At this point, I again wondered if I had not opened up a larger can of worms than I had intended and if I had done the right thing. It was too late now, and time alone would tell.

I tried to ease things a bit. "I want you all to know that if it were not for Mom's illness, I would count myself among the most fortunate men in this world. To have a family that offers so much support, understanding, and personal time as you all do is the primary factor that gives me the strength to cope. I appreciate your concern for Mom and me, but after having attended a few meetings at the support group, I realize that I do not have to look very far to find people who have things far worse than I do. Many of these people handle things just as well as you say I do, if not better. I am not sure what the future holds, how bad things may become, or what difficult decisions I may have to make. I do know that I will be able to handle whatever fate has in store for me with the aid and the love that you and your families have always shown to Mom and me."

"We love you and Mom, Dad," Jil said.

"We love all of you too," I answered.

It was a very poignant moment for all of us.

Terry opened her eyes, sat up, and stretched. She saw us sitting around her and immediately flashed us one of her lovely smiles. It was impossible for us not to smile back.

"Hi, Hon," I said. "Did you have a nice nap?"

A Typical Day

When I was a young man, struggling to make a living for my family, it seemed like I had become a slave to the alarm clock. I would groan in anguish as I rolled over each morning to find the darned button that would silence that horrible clanging noise.

Wonderful visions of a world without alarm clocks danced their way through my thoughts. Imagine being able to sleep as long as I wanted to every morning, ten o'clock, eleven o'clock, even noon if I so desired. I would rise and stagger into the bathroom while I contemplated how glorious life would be if this dream ever turned into a reality. Perhaps when I grew older and had made my mark in life I could retire, and then my dream would come true at last.

Alas, it was not to be. Age plays some sneaky tricks on us older folks, and I know of very few of us old codgers for whom this dream has come true. Most of us find our eyes snapping open at about six or seven in the morning no matter how late we stayed up the night before.

Regardless of how often Terry may have disturbed my sleep the night before, I cannot sleep late. If I do not detect the fragrance of lilies, or hear organ music, I rise and start my day. I have learned to sleep lightly and am usually aware of it if Terry rises to go into the bathroom. Although I leave a night-light on, she often gets lost and cannot find her way to the toilet. On these occasions, I will get out of bed and lead her in to assist her. I consider myself fortunate that she will wake up if she needs the toilet and that we have not had any accidents lately.

On two nights in a row, some time ago, she did have an accident in bed. It appeared to me that this might be evolving into a trend, and I feared she was becoming incontinent. I decided the best thing to do was to purchase a package of Depends for her to wear at night. She hated them to the extent that she somehow managed to control herself at night and overcome her problem. She has not had an accident since, which is something her doctor and I find quite unbelievably amazing, but it really is true.

For a while she was having hallucinations at night. The first time it happened, she woke me up to tell me there was a strange man at the foot of our bed. My eyes sprang wide open, and the hairs on the back of my neck stood up. I was ready to do battle. Of course, there was no one there. I turned on the lights to reassure her that she was just dreaming and that all was well. That first time was quite an eerie sensation. At other times she would see her mother at the foot of the bed and talk to her. Other times she would hear a baby crying and get up to console it. "Don't cry, sweetheart, I'll find your mommy for you," she would say.

At other times she would be certain that there was a close friend of ours standing outside our bedroom window trying to get in. "Let her in," Terry would say, "you know how easily she gets lost." Sometimes I would awaken to find her waving at some imaginary person in the middle of the night. She has no recollection of these happenings the next day and does not believe me if I am foolish enough to tell her about them. I pass it off and do not push it.

There were times when calming her down took quite a while, and I could not get back to sleep. I was tired all the time, and I turned to Terry's doctor for a possible solution. She recommended a drug called Risperdal, and the hallucinations miraculously stopped. Fortunately the drug did not prevent her from awakening at night if she had to use the bathroom. I had feared this might be a side effect. I stopped the Risperdal after about two weeks and found she no longer seemed to need it. Occasionally the hallucinations would return, and I would resume the drug for a few days, which seemed to work fine.

The Alzheimer's, or possibly the medication she has to take, as I have mentioned before, seems to have caused Terry to require more sleep than she used to. She does not usually rise in the morning until I go into the bedroom and waken her. Mornings are a relaxing and pleasant time of the day for me. Terry is still sleeping quietly, and I am content knowing she is at ease and resting comfortably.

We have a cat we call Fernando. He was named after the old-time movie star Fernando Lamas. You may remember that he was the actor who used to say "You look marvelous, my darling" to all the women and "It is better to look good than to feel good."

Every morning Fernando would be right there to greet me and rub against my ankles as I walked into the kitchen. I would bend down to give him a little caress, and he always rewarded my effort with a small muted "meow."

My first order of business is to take care of his needs as he weaves between my feet, watching everything I do and making sure that what I am doing is done correctly and to his liking. Terry and I have always enjoyed having pets, both cats and dogs, and I now find that he is a great source of companionship for me. Actually I brought him into our home because I had read somewhere that having a pet has a calming effect on many people. It does seem that Fernando has a relaxing effect on Terry when he climbs onto her lap and proceeds to softly purr as she caresses him.

I put on a robe and go outside to pick up the newspaper that awaits me in my driveway. I then come in and quickly scan the headlines. I will read the entire paper later on, but first I enjoy doing the crossword puzzles while I am able to concentrate without interruption. I try to keep a steady routine so that everything will seem familiar to her. I start coffee about seven thirty in the morning and prepare something simple for our breakfast. I try to get her up about 8:00 a.m. and start her day off by "trying" to sing a little song to the old tune of "Lazy Mary." It goes something like this. "Lazy Terry, will you get up, will you get up, Lazy Terry, will you get up so early in the morning."

I hear her giggle, and I know she is awake. I do not always go in to get her right away, and if I do not, it will not be long before she comes staggering out of the bedroom. Sometimes she is not quite awake and is a little lost and confused.

"Where are you?" she will call out.

I go into a different routine, and this time I sing another old song called "Someone's in the Kitchen with Dinah."

"I'm in the kitchen with Dinah," I sing.

"And what are you doing?" she may respond if it is one of her good days.

"I'm strumming on the old banjo."

She has probably found me by now, and I continue to sing the old song hoping she will be awake enough this morning to join in. Sure, it sounds crazy, but she is laughing and happy. I have tried to stimulate her, and it has put us both in a good mood. I walk over to her and take her in my arms to give her a little hug and a peck on the cheek.

"I bet you think I love you," I say. "Boy, have I got you fooled."

She laughs knowing I am kidding her, and sometimes, if I am lucky she will think to answer me with an "I love you too." It's a nice way to start the day. I take her by the hand and lead her over to the counter where I have laid out her medication and vitamins. She stares at the counter but cannot find the pills. I hand her a glass of juice and pop the pills in her mouth one by one as she sips the juice and swallows them down. She gives me a big smile and tells me, "That was delicious."

Once again I take her by the hand, and this time I lead her over to the kitchen table where breakfast is waiting. She reacts the same way at every meal. Everything I feed her is delicious to her, and she is always so grateful.

"Look at this, look at this," she exclaims. "It looks wonderful."

This morning it is simply a bowl of cold cereal with sliced fruit and milk. She cannot find the spoon, so I put it in her hand. She sits there not moving.

"Should I eat?" she asks.

I tell her to go ahead, and she lifts the spoon to her mouth.

I sit down across from her, and I start to eat too. I have to watch her and coax her, or she will stop eating and stare into space until I say something to her. At this point in time, she is still capable of feeding herself for most of the meal. As the bowl empties, it becomes more difficult for her to find the food. I move over and sit down next to her so that I can finish feeding her until the bowl is empty.

"Open up," I say, and she opens her mouth childlike.

"Last spoonful," I tell her. "You did great, and I'm proud of you."

She smiles with pleasure.

I pour her coffee for her and tell her it is in front of her. She stares at it unseeingly. I place her fingers around the cup handle, and she starts to sip the coffee. I will have to tell her several times that the coffee is in front of her until she is finished.

"Would you like some more coffee?" I ask.

"No, thank you," she answers.

"I think I would like a little more," I tell her.

"Okay, then I'll have some more too," she said.

I do the dishes while she sits quietly at the table. When I am done, I once again take her by the hand and suggest we go brush our teeth. I fill a cup for her to rinse her mouth with and put toothpaste on her toothbrush. I place the brush in her hand, and she stands there not knowing what to do.

"Should I brush?" she asks, and I tell her to go ahead. Sometimes she cannot find her mouth, and I have to guide the brush to her mouth. While she brushes, I make the bed.

I walk back into the bathroom and tell her she can stop now. I take the toothbrush away from her and rinse the toothpaste off. I hand her the glass of water to rinse her mouth with, and she pours it over her hands. I refill the glass and guide it to her mouth.

"Swish the water around in your mouth and spit it out," I tell her.

She obediently does as I ask, and I wash her face and hands with a face cloth and dry her off.

"Sit on the bed while I brush my teeth and shave, and then we will shower."

I am fortunate that she is so docile and willingly does as I ask. A short time ago, I went into the shower after she had already showered first and noticed that the soap was dry. The next time she showered, I peeked in on her and discovered that she was unable to find the soap. She was just rinsing off with water and not soaping down. I tried to reach in to help her, but this was very awkward, and water was coming out onto the bathroom floor. I soon realized that the best and easiest way to help her get clean was to get in the shower with her.

Sex is a subject that is tastefully and well covered in the various books on Alzheimer's that I have read, and I have no intention of delving into it on a personal level. Suffice to say that most of what I have read is of the opinion that while sex can be a problem in many cases of dementia, it can also be one of the good remaining things left for a couple who both still find enjoyment in it. For many it is a moment to be close again, to feel young again, and to possibly be in love again.

We step out of the shower, and I dry us both off. I sit her on the bed and ask her to raise both feet off the ground so I can slip her panties on. I have to do this because if she tries to do this herself she will either put them on backward, inside out, or with both legs in one leg hole. Next I hold up her bra and ask her to hold up her arms so I can slip the loops over them. I then reach behind her so I can fasten the snaps. The socks come next, and I ask her to lift one foot at a time so that I can slip them on for her. If she tries to do it herself, it is a fifty-fifty chance that she will put the heel on top of her foot and the socks will not go on right. Slacks and shoes go on next, and then I get her to step into her shoes. She is now dressed, and I guide her into the bathroom and place a comb in her hand. She just stands there.

"Comb your hair," I tell her, and she tries to do so. She does this pretty well and I just have to smooth out a few spots.

"Here is your lipstick." I let her try to apply it herself, and she does one side of her upper lip but does not know what to do next. I take the lipstick away from her and finish the other side of her lip.

"Rub your lips together so you can get your lower lip covered." She does so.

"You look marvelous, my darling," I tell her in my best Fernando Lamas impersonation.

She was never vain, but now she stands smiling and admiring herself in front of the mirror like a little girl. She feels pretty and is pleased with herself.

Some of the things she does and says in her confusion are occasionally a bit humorous, For example, one morning she got ahead of me while I was dressing her. The phone rang, and I was distracted for a few moments while I answered it. When I came back, she had put her blouse on inside out.

I smiled. "You have your blouse on inside out," I told her.

She walked over to the mirror and looked at herself.

"Yeah," she said, "but it really doesn't look that bad, does it?"

I had to laugh and told her that I thought it would look even better if we put it on the right way. She laughed with me and agreed.

I do my household chores such as doing a wash, dusting, or working in the garden while it is cool. Some mornings I take her down to the beach for a walk so we can get some exercise. We stroll hand in hand and enjoy looking at the sailboats passing by and watching the bathers swim and play in the waves.

She really loves it when I take her to the local mall and she can browse and do some window-shopping. Everything she sees is beautiful to her, and she oohs and aahs as we look at the different window displays. She gets excited as a little kid if we see something she really likes and I buy it for her. By the time we get home, she will have forgotten I bought it for her, and when I unwrap it and show it to her, she is thrilled all over again.

On the days we go food shopping at the supermarket, I try to keep an eye on her. I hold her hand because she can lose me in a heartbeat and become frightened. Sometimes I get a little careless and I will let her hand go in order to read the label on a can or for some other reason and she will disappear. Usually when she finds herself alone, she will stay put and wait for me to come back and find her.

She has on occasion walked up to someone and told them she is lost and does not know who she is with. There was one occasion when she was confused enough to take some other gentleman's arm, thinking it was me. I had just spotted her as this was happening, and the stunned expression on his face as this attractive woman seemingly accosted him should have been caught on candid camera. It was hilarious, but I managed to contain myself when I walked up to him and just gave him a wink and a smile. I told him it was all right, and he caught on right away. The relief on his face almost caused me to laugh out loud, but I managed to hold it in.

I have always been quick to notice she is gone and been able to find her before whoever she has spoken to panics. They say you don't stop laughing because you grow old. You grow old because you stop laughing.

It is not unusual to see couples our age holding hands while they walk together, but on a few occasions, we have received some rather thoughtless remarks. One woman thought she was being funny when she remarked that when you saw a couple our age holding hands it usually meant one of them had Alzheimer's. Her smile disappeared when I told her that she had no idea how true that statement was in our case. She murmured an "Oh! I'm so sorry" and walked away with tears in her eyes. It was a reflex answer on my part, and I probably should have just let her remark slide. She was just trying to be funny and really meant no harm. "It's all right," I called after her, but she shook her head and kept walking, obviously deeply embarrassed.

I was annoyed and felt my Latin blood rise when another old guy sitting with his friends noticed we were holding hands. "Isn't love grand," he very snidely remarked.

I stopped in my tracks and turned to face him.

"How the hell would someone like you know anything about love," I asked.

His face blanched, and he was speechless as I walked away holding Terry's hand. His friends just sat quietly.

For the most part people just nod and smile pleasantly as we walk by. I am certain that the thought that I am holding her hand because of Alzheimer's does not enter most of their minds. They just view us as a nice old couple who are still in love.

When we have completed our shopping, I push the cart out into the parking lot and open the car trunk to place the groceries in it.

"Should I get in it?" she asks.

"No, hon, you ride up front with me."

She is so cooperative that had I said yes I have no doubt she would have tried to climb into the trunk.

Lunchtime is approaching by the time we get back home, and I will probably prepare something simple like a tuna sandwich, grilled cheese with tomatoes and bacon, or soup with Ritz crackers. I will put an apron on her while she eats. This cuts down on the wash if she should spill something on herself and prevents me from having to change her blouse.

After lunch I do the dishes, and we go into the family room to watch a little TV. It was now apparent that with Terry's ailment it had become impossible for us to take any future vacations. I decided to make our unavoidable confinement as comfortable and pleasant as I possibly could. The new large flat-screen plasma TVs were coming out then, and although they were quite expensive, I rationalized that the money I would spend buying one of them was no more than we would spend on a vacation. It was a good decision because not only was it enjoyable for me but also Terry seemed to focus better on it than she had on the smaller screen we had before.

We both get sleepy after lunch, and it is not unusual for us to doze off while watching TV. She seems to nap longer than I do, which gives me the opportunity to get on my computer and amuse myself by working on this book. I guess it is good therapy for me because it keeps my mind occupied and makes me think. As I mentioned, Terry sleeps more now, and I can get quite a bit of writing done while she does. If I try to work while she is awake, and doing something that does not include her, she is prone to getting cranky and difficult. She has difficulty sitting still too long, and her mind sometimes wanders. She will ask me again who I am, and now she often tells me she wants to go home.

"This is where we live, this is our home. I am your husband and we have three children."

"No, no, this is not my home," she answers fearfully.

It took me a while to figure out that the home she was talking about was the one she lived in with her parents when she was a young girl.

"It's all right, hon, don't you remember you moved away from that home when we got married. That home is way up in New York, and we live here in Florida now."

A glimmer of recollection seems to come to her.

"Is that true?" she asks skeptically.

"It sure is, we have been married a long time, and we still love each other."

She smiles, but she does not answer. At least she seems to be calm again, and I realize she may have already forgotten what she asked me a few moments ago.

The kitchen is a room that Terry and her parents had declared off-limits for me. Terry was a great cook as were her parents, Grandpa Ray and Grandma Ann. The kitchen to me was a mysterious place from which delightful and enticing aromas emanated, and any attempt on my part to assist or even enter this mystic domain of theirs was greeted with gales of laughter. I would walk away slightly miffed.

Actually I knew this was a pretty good deal for me, and I very much enjoyed the fruits of their labor. Unfortunately I found myself in a bit of a dilemma when Terry reached the point where cooking was just too confusing for her to attempt any longer. I realized that if we were to survive, I was now forced to learn the mysteries of the kitchen that had so long been denied me.

I am proud to announce that I have actually learned to boil water without burning it. Seriously, the truth is that I have learned to prepare several simple but delicious meals and to my surprise actually find enjoyment in doing so. I will match my baked salmon, pork tenderloin, or chicken marsala against anyone's. Yeah, I guess I am bragging a little, but I am kind of proud of myself.

Perhaps it may seem odd to you, even a bit crazy, considering how lost and confused she is at times, but Terry can still function in company to some degree. I refuse to give up trying to stimulate her, and I try to give her, as well as myself, the opportunity to find some enjoyment in life. As I mentioned before, she does seem to enjoy being with people and, as many others with her ailment do, often rises to the occasion and does not seem too confused. Tonight there is a dinner dance at one of the local fraternal organizations, and I do not have to cook. We will once again sit at a table with our friends and have a few laughs. One of the better local bands is playing tonight, and although Terry can no longer do all the dance steps she once knew, she can still follow me if I keep it simple. She does seem to manage to have a good time.

If I notice that she is showing any signs of tiring or beginning to act a little too confused, I will give our friends a wink and say good night. I will escort her out to our car and open the car door for her to get in. What I once did because I was trying to be a gentleman has now become a necessity because I know she cannot find the car door handle and will grope for it as though she was blind. I help her into the car and fasten her safety belt for her. Sometimes when she is tired, she is unsure of how to get into the car, and I have to prompt her with a few simple directions such as, "Slip your left leg into the car and put it in front of your seat." I hold her while she does this so she does not lose her balance. "Now move over and sit down on the seat." I have my hands on her shoulders as I help guide her in, and I make sure her fingers are clear when I shut the door.

"Are you sure you know where I live?" she wonders.

It is a question that I have become used to. Notice that she said where she lives, not where we live. Once again I try to explain to her that we are married and that we live in the same house together. She appears a little confused and a little frightened, but she says nothing.

We drive home, and once again she breathes a sigh of relief and is amazed when we pull into our garage. We walk into the house, and Fernando is waiting to greet us by rubbing himself against our ankles again and letting out a few welcoming meows. He is familiar to Terry, and seeing him puts her further at ease. I let her fuss over him for a few minutes, and then I gently steer her into the bedroom and help her prepare for bed.

"Why do I have to take my bra off?" she asks.

She is still not sure I am her husband, and she is modest. I find it odd that she has no objection to my getting in the shower with her, but every night she resists taking her bra off.

"Well, I want to put your nightgown on you, and I'm sure you don't want to sleep with your bra on, right?"

She looks a little skeptical but allows me to remove it.

We brush our teeth. She is tired, and it is late enough for her to go to bed. I help her to slip under the covers. She is almost asleep before her head hits the pillow. I kiss her good night and say, "Good night, hon, I love you." She answers me with a little murmur.

A Moment Of Weakness

My eyes slowly opened, and I turned my head so that I could read the digital numbers on my alarm clock. It was only a little after six in the morning, and Terry had only disturbed me twice last night. I knew I was slept out, and after lying there for a few minutes, I decided that there was just no sense in fighting it.

It was winter, and the room was pitch-black when I rolled out of bed wide awake. I was greeted with the familiar sensation of Fernando's furry body brushing against my legs. I did not turn on the light in the bedroom in order not to wake Terry too early. I found my robe behind the bedroom door, and I groped my way in the darkness to turn on the light in the kitchen.

I went into my usual routine of going out to the driveway to get my newspaper, feed the cat, and then lay out our medications. I put the coffee on and sat down to relax and do my crossword puzzles until it was time to wake Terry. I would wait a while before preparing breakfast so it would be fresh when I woke her to come out into the kitchen and eat. It was my daily quiet time, and I was once again able to relax and feel at ease.

I let my mind wander back to yesterday when I had spent the morning playing golf and afterward sat down to a nice lunch with my friends. I had arranged for the agency to send someone over to stay with Terry while I played golf, and I had been content that she was safe and well cared for.

There were usually about twelve of us, and most of the men were in their fifties or sixties. They liked to kid me that they wanted to be just like me when they grew up. I am the oldest golfer in the group, and while my game has suffered to some extent with age, I am still competitive.

We would push a few tables together, sit down to enjoy lunch, and pay off our bets. There was much complaining about missed shots and bragging about the good ones. We enjoyed "breaking each other's chops," and there was a lot of good-natured laughter. It was just the type of respite I needed to unwind from my duties at home.

One of my golf buddies, as often occurred, was thoughtful enough to ask me how Terry was doing. I told him truthfully that she was fading, which was something that was to be expected with Alzheimer's, but fortunately she was still doing fine physically. Some of the other men overheard the conversation and had listened intently to what I had to say. They were good guys and would sympathetically try to give me some encouragement by telling me what a good job I was doing and what a great guy I was.

"We feel for you, Lou, we really do, we don't know how you handle it," they would say with sincere compassion.

This type of thing was not unusual, and although it sometimes embarrassed me, it did help to hear people offer some consolation and to see the sincerity on their faces as they spoke. The problem was that, other than saying thank you, I had difficulty knowing how to respond. Perhaps thank you was enough, but I really wanted to say more so they could be aware of the gratitude I felt for their interest.

I completed my crossword puzzles and laid my pencil down. It was time for me to start preparing breakfast. As I did so, my mind continued to drift back to yesterday and the kind words my friends had bestowed upon me.

I guess that all things considered, I mused egotistically, I really had held up and handled things fairly well. Admittedly, I occasionally had to swallow hard to rid myself of the large lump that sometimes formed in my throat, but I had carefully tried not to allow myself to complain to anyone too often, and I had been able to maintain an apparently cheerful attitude in company that I was not always actually really feeling. Yes, sir, I patted myself on the back, I was one self-controlled and tough cookie.

I had not elaborated all that was going on with Terry when I spoke to my golf buddies. I had kept it short and sweet and just answered their questions. I have found that, although people will politely ask about her, they really do not want me to go too deeply into detail. I did not tell them how Terry is actually on an emotional roller coaster of peaks and valleys.

She has her good days when she peaks, and then at other times she will plunge into a deep valley of confusion.

Unfortunately it is the valleys that are flattening out and growing longer in length. She tries to climb the peaks again, but she never seems to attain the previous heights and soon slides back to where she was again.

It is as though she is living in a constant fog that mercilessly continues to increase in density. At times the sun allows its bright rays to break through for a short time, and for that *magic* moment, she is almost lucid again. These are wonderful times because they make me feel that, at least for that moment, I have her back again.

I cannot in my wildest imagination conceive of what it must be like for her to be this lost. It is impossible for me not to feel some depression when I consider what a rotten way this is for someone to live out the remaining years of their life.

She sleeps a lot now, and I suspect that part of the reason for this is because she is so unaware of everything that goes on around her. I believe that she is just plain bored. She has lost so much, and I just do not have the stamina to keep her constantly occupied and entertained.

Even when we try to visit family, she grows restless and wants to go home. She used to be so pleased when I took her out for dinner and dancing with friends, but now she becomes restless there too and again wants to go home.

She can no longer follow me when we dance, and I cannot lead her into even the simplest of steps. The fun is slowly going out of her life no matter how hard I try to make her happy. Our social life had gradually lessened mainly because I was now worried about how she would behave in public.

I too was bored, and one evening I decided to take a chance by trying to take her out to our favorite restaurant. She did seem to be having one of her good days. We were seated and were leisurely sipping on our cocktails. All seemed to be going well when she suddenly looked over at me and asked who I was. I went into my usual routine.

"I am your husband Louis, and you are my wife, we have been married for many years."

"No, no, you are not my husband," she contradicted me. "My god, what would he think if he saw me in here with you? I should not be here."

I had never seen her this adamant and fearful before, and from the look on her face, I realized that this was one time I was not going to able to pacify her. I called the waiter over and told him I was having a problem and had to leave. He had waited on us before, knew us well, and quickly understood.

"I owe you for the drinks," I said, and bless him, he answered not to worry, they were on the house.

I quickly got her out of there, and I walked her to our car. She balked and would not get into this strange man's car no matter how I coaxed her. I had visions of someone calling the police and telling them there was a man in the parking lot trying to force a woman to get in his car. I knew I could explain the situation to the police if this happened, but I did not relish the thought of having to do so. I finally was able to assure her, after some time, that I would not harm her and that I would take her home to her husband. I had learned how to be able to stay patient and calm and was careful not to do or say anything that might further upset her.

I opened the car door and to my relief was able to help her in without any further resistance from her. I drove us home, and the moment we pulled into the garage, it was as though nothing had happened, and she was fine again. What had happened a short time ago was completely gone from her memory.

That little episode was pretty much the end of our social life because I never know when she will have another spell like this and create a scene. We no longer go out to eat, and I have given up our dance nights. The noise of the music she once enjoyed so much now seems to confuse and upset her.

Her appetite seems to be diminishing, and she is losing weight. I try to entice her with her favorite foods, and I keep plenty of her favorite ice cream and cookies in the house. I can usually get her to drink a small bottle of Ensure with her meal to aid in her nutrition. I will ask her if she is hungry, and even when she says yes, she does not want to eat when I try to feed her. What she might enjoy today, she will refuse tomorrow. On occasion she will start to eat again, and she might even gain a little weight, but the appetite and weight gains are short-lived.

People in the support group who have gone through the same experience with their loved ones have told me that this could be a sign that she will stop eating altogether. They hint that we might possibly be reaching the end of the line. I have made my children aware of this and have told them that if this is true, then perhaps it is better if she does go before me. They have their own family responsibilities, and I do not want to burden them with the responsibilities involved in taking care of her.

My children understood my thinking, but they had been doing some thinking too and had some different ideas of their own, ideas that I grudgingly had to admit made sense.

"We understand what you are thinking, Dad, and we hope we have you with us forever, but the reality is that there is no guarantee that you will outlive Mom. People with Mom's illness sometimes go on for many years. Conversely, people such as you who appear to be in good shape can surprise everyone and suddenly be gone. The possibility of Mom outliving you has to be considered. She is beyond the point of any of us being able to care for her properly and, as you say, take care of our own family responsibilities too. We cannot care for her as you do and go to work too. We cannot do all the personal things she requires and that you do for her every day. We certainly do not want to suddenly put her in a completely strange environment where she would feel uncomfortable and possibly become frightened. All emotions aside, let's first try to think of what would be best for Mom and for you."

They had evidently foreseen this day coming and had done some research on their own. They had found an excellent facility nearby that offered day care in a secure and professional atmosphere that was both safe and entertaining. If the day ever came when I could no longer care for Terry because of age, illness, or even death, then at least she could go to a place where she was familiar with both the surroundings and the people. They urged me to give respite day care a try and see how it worked out.

I knew they were right, but I was still hesitant. I was certain no one could take care of her like I could, and I guess I felt guilty that I was somehow deserting her. Still, I could not deny that what they were suggesting had a great deal of merit to it, and I finally agreed to try it out for two days a week from nine to three. I was certain that it would not work out and that she would feel lost and be constantly looking for me.

I made arrangements with the assisted living facility they had chosen and dropped her off without any fuss. I stayed home the first day we tried it and sat by the phone waiting for the call I was certain was sure to come.

"Come and get her," they would say. "She is despondent without you, and we cannot console her." That phone call never came.

I went to pick her up at three o'clock and found a happy, smiling Terry who had evidently had a good time. In a way I felt betrayed and hurt to think she could possibly get along without me to guide her, but the truth was they could keep her busy all day long and entertain her much better than I could. I shook it off, and I soon got over it. Our children were right, and I am glad now that I listened to them. Should some mishap befall me that required her to be placed there full-time, the transition should go considerably smoother as she enters a familiar environment.

I felt I had fought the good fight as hard as I knew how and had done all I could for her, but it was a battle that deep down I knew I could never win. In my thoughts, it was as though I was speaking directly to her. I leaned back for a moment, and I found myself going back in time to the beginning of our life together. In my mind, I spoke directly to her as though she was there listening to me.

"Time had taken its toll on us, honey, and where once our skin was smooth, there are now lines beginning to show. That dark curly hair I loved so much now has a few shades of gray in it. I still remember our first date and how when I found the courage to put my arm around your shoulder, you shyly moved a little closer to me. The lines on your face and the gray in your hair do not matter because in my mind's eye you will always be that lovely young girl I fell in love with so many years ago."

I didn't feel it coming, but suddenly there were tears streaming down my cheeks, and my body began to rack with sobs. I did not know what was happening to me, and I slumped against the wall and slid to the floor as I tried to regain control of myself. I could not stop, and I felt weak. I could not remember ever having wept this hard before in my life. I don't know how long I sat there on the floor, it could not have been for more than a few minutes, but it seemed like an eternity. Slowly the sobs began to subside, and I took my handkerchief out and dried the tears from my face.

I sat there for a few minutes thinking about what had just happened to me. *Yeah*, I thought, *you're some tough cookie*, and I began to mentally chastise myself for my weakness. As I continued to gain control, I began to give it further thought, and it occurred to me that perhaps it was just as well that this had finally happened. I guess I had been holding in a lot of my feelings for quite some time, and I felt like a weight had been lifted off my chest.

I realized then that I was probably far overdue in letting my emotions come out.

I stood up, still struggling for control. It was time to get Terry up, and I slowly walked over to the bedroom door. It took quite some effort, but I managed to sing my usual little wakeup song to her.

"Lazy Terry, will you get up, will you get up, Lazy Terry, will you get up so early in the morning?"

I found I could still smile when I heard her cute little giggle.

Where Did The Years Go?

*Y*es, where have the years gone? It seems impossible, but it has been six years since I wrote the previous chapter, and as closely as I can estimate, it has been twenty-two long years since Terry showed her first signs of Alzheimer's. Much has changed in this time span, and I have learned many things pertaining to human nature and the effect this horrific disease can have on those compassionate souls we call caregivers.

In twenty-two years, I have traversed the many slippery and rocky plateaus Alzheimer's has caused me to stumble upon. I say stumble because, try as I might, I know mistakes were made. I call them plateaus because in most cases it seems the disease flattens out for a while and then takes a sudden drop to an even lower level.

I want to share with you a few of my experiences and some of the lessons I have learned as the years have passed by. It is my hope that perhaps those of you who are beginning to go through similar experiences will profit from what I have to tell you and learn you are not alone.

I want to share the story of how fate has directed my life, given me hope, and has gradually made me whole again. I do so because I want others to understand that with the proper attitude, life can become good again.

I know the beginning of my tale may seem somewhat disheartening and disturbing to you, but as you continue, you will begin to see how, regardless of adversity, it is possible for anyone's life to change for the better. Nothing in life really ever stays the same. For better or for worse, it is up to you.

Alzheimer's has continued to take its course on Terry through the years. Terry is completely oblivious to all that is around her, and it has become very disheartening for me to visit with her. Try as I might, she offers absolutely no response to anything I say or do. Suddenly, after months of silence, an unexpected and heartwarming miracle takes place. She may open her eyes for a few seconds and seem to focus on me, or even respond with a "Yeah" to a question I may have asked. I cannot help but feel elated, for in that brief moment, it is almost like she is back with me again. That is what I, and many of my fellow caregivers, call "the magic moment."

If it is a simple reflex, or she is trying to actually answer, this I do not know. She is incontinent and completely helpless and no longer knows who I am or who her children are. She sits in her wheelchair, eyes closed, and is usually slumped over. She often becomes agitated and wrings her hands while she moans. Oddly enough, her earlier loss of appetite disappeared, and now her one joy in life seems to be eating. Her appetite is good, although she does not put on weight. Those who, with the best of intentions, had tried to prepare me for the worst as she lost weight would be quite surprised to see her still here, and eating so well.

There are plateaus for the caregiver too, and as the years go by, they also level off for a while. We learn to adjust to the new lower level our loved one has fallen to, and hopefully, we rise to a higher level of understanding and admission as to what we are feeling. I have finally reached the very bitter realization that the wife I once knew and loved, the mother my children once knew and loved, no longer exists. Yes, she still breathes, but everything that made her the person that she once was is gone. All that exists for us now are the memories of a wonderful woman and mother, and our desire to keep her well cared for and as comfortable as possible. We will always love her.

Allow me, at this point, to continue from where I left off in the last chapter and fill you in on what has transpired since then.

I held on to her and kept her at home with me for many years as you know, but as I will explain later on, once again, fate stepped in, and the painful decision to let her go was made for me. One day was pretty much like the other, and it was a very dull way to live. There was little pleasure in life. The highlight of our existence, as you have read earlier, was when our family came to visit and tried to cheer us up. Terry seemed to be able to respond to some degree when the family visited, and that pleased us all. My son-in-law continued to come over on Sundays to watch football on TV with me. A weekly game of golf with my son was also one of my few pleasures. My daughter was constantly on the phone or dropping by. Friends would phone occasionally but did not visit. Most preferred to remember Terry the way she used to be. They slowly drifted away. I understood, and I could hardly blame them. We were not pleasant company to be around.

Every day about 3:00 p.m. she would start to pace. She would get up from where she was seated and walk into the kitchen, around the partition, and into the dining room, back into the family room where she had been seated, and repeat the process over and over, again and again and again. The doctor called it twilight syndrome and prescribed some medication to calm her down. It helped to some degree.

As the days dragged by, I started to have the same dream almost every night. I would dream that I walked through an entrance into a poorly lit room. As my eyes became accustomed to the light, I noticed that the walls were made of solid concrete. I felt very uncomfortable and I turned to go back out. I suddenly became frightened when I realized the door had disappeared. I looked for another way out, a window perhaps, or a stairway, but there was no way out. I would wake up in a cold sweat and reach out in bed to find Terry. I would feel some comfort when I felt her next to me and knew she was all right.

I had told myself that I would accept the responsibility that had been thrust upon me with as much grace and love as I could muster. Up until now I thought I had done pretty well. Unfortunately, it did not take a psychiatrist for me to figure out that subconsciously, and after all these years, I felt trapped.

This made me feel guilty. Even though I realized I had no control over my subconscious, I felt I was somehow mentally deserting her. I thought I was stronger than that, but the emotional stress of constantly trying to be alert to her needs was wearing me down. As I mentioned, I had had moments of some depression before but had always been able to perk myself up. This was the strongest wave of depression that had ever swept over me, and it frightened me. Was this then how I would spend my remaining days? I lamented.

This, I knew, was not a good attitude, and I grudgingly began to sense that perhaps I needed more help. It is difficult to understand for anyone who has not experienced being an Alzheimer caregiver, the stress such a responsibility can put on even the strongest person.

The support group I had mentioned earlier met once a month. They were helpful, but if I missed a meeting, it would be two months before I would be able to attend a meeting again and hopefully get some help.

A friend, who was also a caregiver, mentioned another group that met every Monday morning from 9:30 a.m. to 11:00 a.m. He said he was attending their meetings. He said he felt that they were quite good and had helped him quite a bit. After a short period of procrastination, I decided to give them a try.

I arranged for the woman who helped me with Terry to come in on Mondays so I could attend the group meetings. Going to this support group turned out to be one of the best decisions I have ever made. Meeting once a week offered a far superior and explicit method of counseling than the first group had, and I found a greater understanding of what Alzheimer's was really all about.

As I listened, I felt more and more comfortable with my own thoughts and emotions. I learned I was not so different from anyone else. I was now among people who had walked, or were walking, in the same shoes I was. We understood each other like no one else possibly could. Confidences that whoever was speaking thought they could never express in an open meeting came out. They were accepted with compassion, understanding, and usually with some very good advice. There was a strong sense of trust, and we knew that everyone listening had an honest desire not to criticize, but to help.

The New Support Group

I think it might be beneficial if I gave everyone a closer look at what can transpire at a good support group meeting. Hopefully it might inspire someone to search out a support group near them and possibly do themselves a big favor by joining.

My friend had told me the support group meetings were held at a local community center close by that I was familiar with. I arranged for Terry to be taken care of, and at nine, I drove over and parked my car in their lot. I walked in through the front entrance, looked around for a moment, and soon found the room where the group met. I walked into the room, and just as had occurred with the first support group, I was quickly approached and welcomed by a very friendly and pleasant woman. I was asked to write my name and phone number down on an attendance list, and she showed me how to make out a name tag for myself.

I was a bit early, and there were not many people present as I sat down. Those that were present all wore name tags too, and most greeted me with a friendly smile. Some even read my name tag and said, "Hi, Lou." This surprised me because the people at the other support group had been slightly reticent. This was probably because by meeting only once a month we did not have the opportunity, or time, to really get to know one another.

The room began to fill as more people walked in. At nine thirty the doors were closed for privacy, and I learned that, like Las Vegas, what was said in here, stayed in here.

A well-spoken and pleasant-looking gentleman stood before the group and started the meeting. He introduced himself as the president of the group and welcomed everyone. He then asked any newcomers to please raise their hands. I happened to be the only newcomer on this particular day, and he asked me to stand up, introduce myself, and tell them who I was caring for. I did so and sat back down.

He continued on, explaining that after the meeting those of us who were free to make it meet at a certain nearby restaurant for lunch to relax and that everyone was invited. He further informed us that we met as a group at a different restaurant every Thursday, and that the person we were caring for was invited too. Alzheimer's was not discussed at these dinners, and it was intended to be a social evening out. (Perhaps for some, myself included, it would be their only social evening out if they could free themselves to come. I did not see how I could make it at this time because I was hesitant about asking anyone to watch Terry in the evenings.) He assured us that no one would be concerned about the inflicted one's manners or behavior. Everyone understood.

One of the facilitators stood up and informed everyone where we were dining this Thursday, and a sign-up list was passed around so she would know how many reservations had to be made.

Another woman stood up and announced that a one-day bus outing was being planned for a nearby destination, and another sign-up list was passed around. I happily realized that this group not only offered counseling, but also a social life to help overcome loneliness. All this took only a few minutes, and when no one had any further announcements to make, it was time to get down to business.

There were two Alzheimer's Association certified facilitators, and although it was not a prerequisite for certification, both were registered nurses. One facilitator had lost her husband to Alzheimer's, and the other was still a caregiver. On this day, there were twenty people present. The facilitators split the group in half in order to make it possible for everyone to have a chance to speak. The meetings usually lasted about an hour and one half, or slightly longer if needed. A sliding partition was used to split the room, and in this case, one facilitator and ten people were on either side.

As with the earlier support group, I sat there listening with interest as the first person was called upon to tell her story and describe how things were going in her life. She told of the experiences and the problems she was having, who it was she was caring for, how far along they were, and how long she had been caring for her loved one.

Some were caring for a spouse, others for a parent, a sister or a brother, or even just a friend. The facilitator would offer advice, and other members would speak up occasionally with additional suggestions they hoped might help. As in the prior support group, there almost always seemed to be someone who had experienced a similar problem, and they would share their experience on what they thought they had done right, or perhaps even wrong. What they felt they had done right often offered solutions, what they felt they had done wrong often prevented mistakes. Their input was invaluable.

I was surprised, and very impressed, when I discovered that almost half the people present were survivors who had already lost their loved ones. It was explained to me, when I asked, that the reason they kept coming back to the meetings was because they felt the support group had helped them so much. They had the unselfish desire to pay back and to use their experience as a way of giving something back to others for what they felt had been done for them. To me, this attitude spoke volumes about the support group. They too were exceedingly helpful in their advice.

As I listened to the others relate their experiences, and heard as before the many similarities to my own experiences, I began to feel slightly less alone. I had, of course, known from the first group, that others were in the same boat as I, but somehow, the way these people openly verbalized their problems, apparently holding nothing back if they thought they could help someone with a problem really impressed me. A wave of sympathy swept through me because I realized that compared to some of the stories I was hearing, perhaps I did not have it too bad after all.

Some related their stories and problems in a very controlled manner, keeping a tight rein on their feelings. Some of the stories told were about humorous antics their charge might have performed. A little laughter was good and served to ease some of the tension that anyone might be feeling. Others became quite emotional, and tears flowed freely. Gender did not matter, and both men and women occasionally lost control. No one thought any less of them at these moments. Indeed, it had also happened to most everyone present at one time or another. There were times when someone would come in that was very set in their ways. They were skeptical about most of what they were hearing, sometimes very much in denial and slightly argumentative about the suggestions that were made to aid them. They were difficult to get through to, and a few would often not return.

Conversely, as time went by, many would eventually realize that their way was not working and return with a different attitude. All were listened to with sincere compassion and interest. Let me give you just a few examples of some of the stories that were told.

One woman told of how her gentle and docile husband of many years had become very aggressive and broken several of her ribs. As I already had been told, the afflicted ones had no control over their behavior.

Another woman told of how her husband, who did not seem to be too far along and seemed capable of still driving, went out to buy a newspaper. He was gone for hours, and in desperation she finally called the police.

He had gotten confused, made a wrong turn, and just kept driving. They eventually found he had driven from central Florida all the way up to Tallahassee in northern Florida. An Alzheimer's patient can go from perfectly lucid to completely confused in seconds.

We all had to laugh at the next story because, although I am sure it was not funny at the time it happened, it was now told with humor. This woman's husband was accustomed to sleeping in the nude. He did not seem too far along in his affliction, and he liked to sleep late, usually until eleven in the morning. One morning, while he was still sleeping, she decided to make a quick visit to the grocery store. She was certain she would be back before he awoke. When she returned home, she found their son, who worked nearby, standing at the front door. "Mom," he said, "we have to talk."

It seems this was the day that the lawn man cut their grass. The lawn mower must have awoken her husband, and being a sociable man, he walked outside to greet them, still in the nude. Fortunately the lawn people knew of the situation and where his son worked. They called the son, and he got his dad back into the house. It was a lesson learned, and she did not leave him alone again.

One woman smiled as she told us her story. Her husband was in a nursing home, and she went to visit him. He greeted her with a big, happy smile. "Good news," he said as he informed her that he was getting married. She responded that that was nice, but he was already married to her, and she was his wife. "No, no" he said, "You're not my wife, but you are invited to the wedding." When asked what his new bride's name was, he did not know, "But we hold hands all the time," he said.

It is not an unusual occurrence for patients who have Alzheimer's to become attracted to each other in the nursing homes. Some have to be watched pretty closely. Most caregivers understand that the patient is not aware of what they are doing and take no offense. At first, it may cause some pain to the spouse, but eventually the usual reaction is to just laugh it off and be glad the patient had found some happiness that is really actually harmless.

The facilitator had waited a while to get to me in order to give me a chance to get used to the group and the way they operated. She finally turned to me and asked if I would like to speak. I was advised that I did not have to speak if I was not ready. She explained that they would be happy to hear what was going on in my life and help if they could, but that nothing was going to be forced.

I hesitated for just a short moment, but I knew if I was to be helped, I had to get involved. I chose to speak and haltingly told my story. A lump formed in my throat as I described some of what I was experiencing with Terry. I told of my sense of loss, and I had to pause a moment before I could continue.

I went home that day, slightly overwhelmed with much of what I had heard. I had been made to feel very comfortable with this group, and I continued to attend every Monday. I learned about the many important legal aspects involved that I was unaware of, particularly the importance of getting the advice of an elder law attorney. I have mentioned the cost of nursing home care earlier and how, with the attorney's help, it is possible to save thousands of dollars in expenses. Any fees you may have to pay the attorney will be more than compensated for in a very short time.

In the course of the meeting, this situation was posed. You are taking a flight to some destination. You have a child or some other helpless person with you. The stewardess instructs the passengers with the usual little speech on emergency procedures. As part of the little speech, the passengers are asked, "Who do you put the oxygen mask on first when they fall down in front of you, yourself or your child?" The answer is to put your own on first. It may sound selfish, but the reason this is what you are told to do is because they do not want you to pass out before you can finish helping the other person. It made perfect sense to me. The point was being driven home once again. If you want to help and give proper care to your loved one, you must first take care of yourself, or you may not be there when you are needed to help.

The facilitators tried to be there every Monday, but there were times when family matters, sickness, or vacations made it impossible for them both to be there. The facilitator who had to take over the entire meeting alone often could not get to everyone so they could speak in the time allotted.

I had been attending meetings for quite some time when I was approached by the steering committee and asked if I would help out as a substitute facilitator. The idea was for me to step in when one of the regular facilitators could not be present and take over a group. I was surprised and flattered at the request, and I was more than happy to comply.

I went to the local Alzheimer's Association chapter for training and am now a certified facilitator. I feel good about what I am doing, knowing I am contributing something by trying to help others. I was surprised when I discovered the unexpected pleasure I derived from what I was doing. I sometimes wondered if I might not actually be gaining more than those I was trying to help. I mentioned this to the other facilitators. They smiled at me and nodded their heads. They knew exactly what I meant. Imagine the exaltation a facilitator feels when someone walks in with tears in their eyes, and you can send them home with a small smile of hope on their face.

The support group became like a second family to most of us, and if someone lost a loved one, most of us attended the service. It was very comforting for both the survivor and their families to see us there, and our presence was always very much appreciated. *Support* was the key word.

While attending many of the services to help comfort a member of the group, I noticed things seemed to be different than at other services I had attended for family and friends in the past. In the past, there was often a very emotional outpouring of uncontrollable grief. Tears would cascade down the faces of relatives, and many a sob could be heard.

With Alzheimer's services, there seemed to be a different attitude. Of course there was grief, and occasionally the tears did flow in abundance, but usually along with that grief was also the survivor's understanding that the person they had loved so well, for so many, many years, was no longer suffering the indignities Alzheimer's had thrust upon them. Often they would admit, with a sad little smile on their faces that in all honesty, and along with the grief, there was also a strong sense of relief. There always seemed to be an abundance of mixed emotions.

The truth actually was that most caregivers had already done their grieving and shed their tears throughout the many years they had sacrificed and cared for their loved ones. Still the loss was great, it was the end of life as they had known it for so many years, and this very confusing thought entered many minds, "What do I do now?"

Murphy's Law

Things were going pretty good. The support group had helped me a great deal, and although things were still not easy, my depression had lessened considerably and I felt much better. That was about to change and Murphy's Law came into effect, "Whatever can go wrong, will go wrong".

It was one of Terry's afternoons for day care at the assisted living facility and I was working around the house trying to tie up some loose ends when the phone rang. It was the A.L.F. calling to inform me that Terry had fallen a few moments ago and seemed to be in pain. They informed me that they needed my permission to call 911 and have an ambulance come to get her.

This type of thing had happened before because they were required to call me if she did something as simple as even scratch herself and they had to put a band aid on the wound. This of course, in at way was at good thing and I appreciated them keeping me informed, but it was usually something of a trivial nature. I would thank them for informing me and let it go at that.

My first reaction was that they were just following procedures and probably over reacting to cover themselves and I asked them to wait until I got there before they called for an ambulance.

My home was only a matter of minutes away and I dropped everything and was there in about ten minutes. My stomach flip flopped, and I felt like someone had punched me, when I saw Terry laying on the floor in an awkward position. They said they had left her there because she was in too much pain when they tried to move her. Upon seeing her laying there, and the pain on her face, I immediately told them to go ahead and call 911.

The small amount of time that had elapsed probably made no real difference, but a sense of guilt overcame me and I felt I had made a mistake and probably should have given them permission to call 911 immediately when they had first called me on the phone.

The paramedics arrived quickly. They managed to get her on a stretcher as gently as possible, and then carefully placed her in the ambulance. I followed them closely in my car to the hospital emergency room, which was packed as most emergency rooms usually are. Fortunately, the position she was in seemed to have eased the pain and she did not seem to be too uncomfortable as she lay on the stretcher.

We waited impatiently for them to see her and eventually she was wheeled away and X-rays were taken of her hip. Sure enough, as we had feared, her hip was broken, and she was scheduled for surgery the next morning. I managed to get in touch with our children and informed them of their mom's condition. One by one they quickly arrived at the hospital to see her and to support me.

The hospital had her records and was aware of her condition and that she had Alzheimer's. The E.M. physician on duty was concerned that she might be incontinent and decided that in order to keep her clean it would be wise to insert a catheter in her. I did not like the idea and suspected it was really done to in an effort to make things easier on themselves. (Her regular doctor had it removed the next day.) She was placed in a semi private room and we all gathered around her and tried to let her know we were there and loved her. They had sedated her and I cannot say if she was aware we were there or not, but we all felt better about just being there.

I feared she would harm herself further if she tried to get up during the night. I thought of asking if there was a private nurse available for hire, but it was late and I really did not feel right about leaving her alone. There was a fairly comfortable looking easy chair in the room and I decided to push it as close to her bed as possible and spend the night there.

As I have told you, I had grown used to sleeping lightly and I was sure I would hear her if she tried to get up. I guess because they had sedated her she slept well and did not move or disturb me. I slept poorly but was glad I had stayed. I was very concerned for her.

The main reason for my concern was because I had heard that hip surgery, at her age, was considered a very dangerous procedure, one that the patient often did not survive. In her case, I am happy to report, everything went well. They started rehab almost immediately, and in a few days she was moved to a nursing home where further rehab was continued. She was very unsure and shy about trying to walk and did not co-operate well. They surmised she was probably afraid of falling again.

After a few weeks of rehab they felt she was not showing any improvement and there was no more that they could do for her. They were ready to release her. She was a dead weight and although I did not want to admit it I had to painfully concede, that at my age, I lacked the physical strength to lift her in and out of bed or do the many other things necessary for he well being. I tried putting a plastic lawn chair in the shower to try and sit her on while I washed her, but just getting her in the chair was at strain.

In all honesty, I don't know if I could have found ways to somehow overcome some of these problems, but I realized that the truth was that, hard as I might try, the nursing home could take much better care of her than I could. I knew I had to overcome my own sense of impending loss, and put what was best for her to the forefront. I had no choice but to place her permanently in the nursing home. Fate, I felt, had made the decision for me and as difficult a decision as it was I knew the time had come to let her go.

Fortunately, I had heeded the advice of the support group and enlisted the aid of a elder law attorney. It had taken me about three months to get my holdings in order so that he could help me apply for Medicaid. I had been warned that this day would eventually come and I was prepared. I never could have afforded to place her in a nursing home where she would get proper care. I don't know what I would have done without it or how I could have survived financially.

The nursing home she was in was considered one of the best in the area. I visited her almost every day and often helped feed her. She was in a wheelchair now, but still seemed to know when I, or our children visited her. She appeared to be comfortable and content for the most part.

There were times when I would stand back and observe what the nurses aides were doing without their being aware I was there. I was pleased to see the compassion they treated, not only Terry, but all their patients with. They would hold a hand, caress someone's hair, adjust them to a more comfortable position and speak soothingly if someone seemed agitated. They seemed to honestly care and the more I saw, the more convinced I became that the correct decision had been made.

Even so, guilt would occasionally creep up on me against all logic. I missed her terribly and there was always a terrible void when sometimes during the night I would reach over in bed to see if she was there and okay. It was something I had become used to doing when she was home and I was caring for her. Half asleep, I would often be shocked to find her missing, and going back to sleep was sometimes a problem.

Depression would return and my mind would race with a million thoughts and memories. Perhaps there was some kind of contraption that would have helped enable me to lift her and care for her I would rationalize. Had I really done the right thing? Fortunately, my family was very supportive and it helped, that they too, agreed that I really had no choice and what I had done was really the best thing for her.

A Small Token Of Kindness

Terry had been gone for about a week, and I sat on my couch wondering what I would do with myself today. As I sat there, I recalled my dream, the one in which I had felt so trapped. It felt so strange to suddenly discover that now I was free. I could go anywhere I wanted, anytime I wanted. Simple things that I had not been able to get away to do for so long, things everyone else takes for granted, were once again within my reach.

The problem was that I was so used to watching over Terry that, crazy as it may seem, I missed taking care of her. I felt like there was a big void in my life. My children all worked and were busy with their own lives. I have no complaints with them, they were very good to me, I was invited to dinner fairly often, and they would phone to check up on me a few times a week to make sure I was okay.

In a way, I found it a bit humorous because it felt like we had reversed roles. They were now the parents, and I was the kid they were worried about and checking up on.

I played golf with the guys and enjoyed the games, but the wisecracking and kidding around was the part I thought was the most fun. I continued to go to the support group meetings and have lunch with them afterward.

The weekly Thursday evening dinners were good too. There were lots of laughter as we kept each other's spirits up. I did odd jobs around the house to keep busy— you know what I mean, the ones we all have a tendency to put off for too long. It was not too long before I had everything shipshape, and I could not help thinking how pleased Terry would have been to see our "honey, do" list completed.

I had been able to stay busy during the days, but the evenings and nights were terribly lonely. Terry was constantly on my mind. I would try to get engrossed watching TV most nights, but my mind would wander. I would sometimes doze fitfully and wake up with a start, looking for her and wondering where she was. I would sadly realize she was no longer with me, and depression would again set in. Eventually I would go to bed and then, tired as I might be, have trouble falling asleep.

I thought about perhaps taking in a movie, and I tried it a few times, but it just wasn't as much fun without someone to nudge with your elbow at the good parts, or discuss some of the scenes with later on. I used to enjoy league bowling, but the season was over, so that was out. Going to a bar to chat with people that had had too much to drink was not my style. I really wanted to find something I could enjoy doing evenings to keep my mind off things, but what?

It was a Tuesday morning when the phone rang. It was an old friend and golf buddy calling to see how I was doing, and of course I downplayed my true feelings and told him things were going great. We chatted for a while about golf and sports, and then he asked if I would like to meet him and his wife at the Italian American Club that evening for dancing and a pasta dinner.

I suspect that he possessed the insight to realize that I probably was quite a bit lonelier than I was letting on. I know now, in retrospect, that he had been leading up to this invitation all along when he called. He said the old gang that Terry and I used to hang out with in the old days, when she was well, would be there and they would love to see me. Terry and I had been part of this group for years until we could no longer socialize. They were the same group we used to go to the Moose Lodge with, as you may recall, and the ladies were the same ones that used to help Terry when she had to go to the ladies' room. Good folks and always fun to be with. I thanked my friend for thinking of me, and I jumped at the chance to be with them again.

"I'll be there with bells on, I'm looking forward to it," I eagerly told my friend.

That evening I pulled into the once-familiar parking lot of the IAC, and a wave of nostalgia coursed through me as I thought of the many times Terry and I had been here. I felt odd, and slightly guilty. What in the world was I doing here without her?

I saw a few familiar faces as I got in line to buy my ticket. We nodded at each other, not quite remembering who the other one was. I walked into the main room and almost immediately saw the table my friends were sitting at. They stood up to greet me, and I was engulfed in a sea of handshakes from the men, and hugs and kisses from the women. I had not expected a welcome like this, and I was deeply moved. In the course of the evening people, I had not seen in years walked over to our table to ask about Terry and to say hello to me. It felt good.

Old times were rehashed. Someone would say, "Do you remember when this or that happened?" and it would start a lively conversation going. It was great to laugh at some of the old memories. I was having a ball. It was just what I needed.

We ate our pasta and meatballs, and the music started. I felt a bit like a fifth wheel at the table and I wished Terry could have been there to dance with me. Many of the ladies present were widows, and I had known their husbands as well as them in the past.

"Why don't you ask some of the ladies to dance, Lou?" my friend suggested, "They all know you and would probably love to have someone to dance with."

It had been a long time since I had danced, but it sounded like a good idea, and I thought, *What the heck, I'll give it a try*. They were playing a nice foxtrot, and I walked over and asked one of the ladies if she would like to dance. She was an old friend also and was happy to accommodate me. She asked about Terry, and we chatted casually as we danced. I danced with a few other ladies that night and recalled, with a little touch of sadness, how much Terry and I had loved to dance together. It was a very pleasant and comfortable evening among old friends. Well, I thought, I had found something to do for at least one evening a week, and Tuesday night at the IAC soon became an enjoyable habit. That evening was the best fun I had had in years.

That night, as I lay in bed the many negative thoughts that usually plagued my mind were replaced with a very pleasant review of the night's events. I even started to mentally review dance steps that I used to be capable of doing with Terry before she could no longer dance. I believe that, for a change, there must have been a smile on my face as I fell asleep that night. It was the best night's sleep I had had in quite a while.

Life takes many twists and turns, and it seems that almost everything we do in life somehow touches someone else's life. My friend probably never knew it, until I finally thanked him one evening. With a simple phone call, and a small token of kindness, my old friend had begun to bring about some very positive changes in mine. I was about to embark on a life that I never would have believed, in my wildest dreams, was possible for someone like me.

Starting A New Life

Tuesday evenings were great. I enjoyed everything about them—the company, the music, and the dancing—but for the rest of the week, the evenings were still very lonely, empty, and depressing.

I desperately wanted to find a way to overcome this. My mind flailed around in all directions looking for an answer, and then, I finally allowed an obvious thought that I had guiltily been suppressing to enter my mind. If one evening out could lift my spirits so much, what would happen if I went out one or two more nights a week? Some people enjoy being alone, I know, they seem to want their space, but I was not one of them.

The more I thought about it, the more the idea appealed to me. I remembered that there were several other places where Terry and I used to go occasionally for an evening of dancing. There were fraternal organizations such as the Elks Club, the Eagles, the Moose Lodge, and the American Legion, to name a few.

Most of them were primarily frequented by couples, but I was aware that there were usually a few single women and men looking for someone to dance with, lonely people like myself, many of whom I believed were only in search of a little companionship, someone to have a few laughs with, perhaps have a dance or two with, and then call it an evening.

I really was not quite all that naive. I knew there would probably be women out there in search of a closer relationship, and I gave that possibility some heavy thought. My intentions were good, and I had no desire to become involved with anyone. I just wanted to make friends, enjoy an evening out, and have a little fun.

I came up with a very simple and obvious solution to avoid what I considered might possibly be a problem. I would just tell everyone the truth, that I was married and my wife was in a nursing home with Alzheimer's.

The plan served two purposes: One, if I did not let them know I was married, they would probably eventually find out I was anyway, and I would be branded a cheat. Two, it would insulate me from any woman with more permanent plans. Being married would certainly place me off-limits, or at least make me considerably less accessible.

Good thinking, I thought, now I had everything covered. I also consoled myself by reasoning, that, certainly, nothing I did at this point in time could possibly cause my wife any pain. She was now almost completely unaware that I even existed.

Saturday morning came, and I woke up thinking about the possibility of finding the courage to go dancing that night. I agonized and vacillated back and forth most of the day. Was this somehow different than going to the IAC where I was among old friends? I wondered if I was just rationalizing and fooling myself. Was I, in a way, actually not being fair to my wife?

On the other hand, I asked myself, did I really think that sitting on the couch and weeping for my wife would, in any way, do her any good? I would do it if I thought it would help, I honestly would, but I knew it really would not help her, or me. It would just hurt my children more to see their dad in pain like that. Actually it was they who encouraged me to get out and find a life.

I deliberately pushed these thoughts out of my mind, and the words to a once-popular old song played over and over in my mind, "Saturday night is the loneliest night of the week."

I ate my dinner in a leisurely fashion that night, and when I was finished, I walked into my bathroom and stood before the mirror. I wondered who that person staring back at me was. Did I know him? I continued to soul search. I was still not sure what I was going to do.

In a zombie-like fashion, I went through the motions. I shaved, showered, and then dressed myself in a neatly casual manner. I tried not to let my mind wander as I entered the garage, got into my car, turned on the ignition, and backed out. There were butterflies in my stomach as I headed for the American Legion Post. I was going to give it a try, and if my guilty conscience caused me to be too uncomfortable, I could always get up and leave.

The parking lot was pretty full, but I found a space. I walked in and heard the music playing. A man at the door stopped me and asked to see my membership card.

I had forgotten about that. I explained that I had belonged long ago but had dropped out some time ago. I turned to leave, and in a way, I was half relieved that fate had intervened, but he stopped me and asked me if I would like to rejoin. I heard myself say "Sure," and he had me fill out an application. I was then allowed to enter as his guest.

The band was pretty good, and the dance floor was filled. I looked around and spotted an empty seat against the rear wall. I continued to glance around the room and tried to relax. It seemed like a good idea for me to try and separate the singles from the couples. I didn't want to get in trouble by asking someone's wife or girlfriend to dance.

There were some pleasant-looking ladies sitting around smiling and laughing, and I struggled to find the courage to ask one of them to dance. I worried about rejection. Suppose they said "No, thank you" and sent me away. I had always been pretty outgoing and certainly not at all shy, but tonight I was as nervous as a teenager going out on his first date.

I tried hard not to show any sign of the turmoil that was going on inside of me. I sat back trying to look at ease and relax. People would walk by and nod. I would smile and nod back. Enough of this, I said to myself, either get up and dance or go home.

With a mind full of misgivings, I stood up and walked over to a table where about five women sat. I smiled and asked one of them if she would like to dance. To my relief, she smiled back, rose from her chair, and walked to the dance floor with me.

"I don't think I have seen you here before," she said as we danced and then told me her name.

"My name is Lou, and yes, it's been a long time since I've been here," I answered.

"How come?" she asked.

"Well, my wife has been ill with Alzheimer's. I took care of her at home for many years until she broke her hip, and I could no longer handle her. She is now in a nursing home, and to tell the truth, this is my first night out on the town, and I'm a little nervous." Honesty, I thought, was the best policy.

That had been easy. She now knew I was married, and she had not walked off the dance floor.

"Oh, Lou! I'm so sorry to hear that. It must have been very difficult for you," she said with compassion.

We chatted along as we danced, and soon the song was over. I walked her back to her table and returned to my seat. I looked over at her table and could see her speaking to the other women seated there. They all had their heads together as they glanced over at me. It was a pretty good guess that by now they all knew my story and that I was married. Mission accomplished, I thought.

I had broken the ice, and asking the next woman to dance was easier. I danced with several women after that and managed to somehow let all of them know I was married. It didn't seem to bother any of them. Perhaps they felt safe with me. Some of them actually thanked me for my honesty. "Most men would have tried to keep the fact that they were married a secret," they said.

I came to the dance again the next Saturday, and many of the same women were there. After a few Saturdays, I had made friends with many of them and was often invited to join them at their table. Most of the ladies were really nice, and we just danced as friends. I was behaving myself very well.

The months passed, and Terry's condition remained the same. She continued to show no response to anything other than opening her mouth for food when a spoon touched her lips.

It was pitiful to realize that although her pulse still beat, to all intents and purposes, she was no longer a part of this world, and she would never ever be able to return to me.

I continued to go dancing and found I could enjoy life again. My depression slowly subsided and was almost gone. I had somehow evolved and placed myself into a world that that was new and exciting to me.

Time went by. My intentions had always been good, but I guess it was inevitable that I would eventually weaken and meet someone special. Someone with whom the chemistry clicked and with whom I was very compatible.

We enjoyed doing the same things, and I was no longer lonely. She too had been a caregiver, and we understood each other very well. It also helped to know, as we met other couples, that we were not at all that unique and that many other couples under similar circumstances had paired off too.

My mind drifted back to the man I had met in the first support group. I was behaving now in the same way he had. I was now walking in the same shoes he had worn, and I was glad I had found the compassion to not judge him too harshly. Who among us knows what fate may have in store for them next.

Life was so simple when I was young. Terry and I would grow old together. We would have family gatherings and watch our grandchildren grow up. We would dine out with friends, and we would take vacations and go on cruises. We would bicker and make up and just enjoy life, loving each other until our time was up.

Never in my wildest dreams did I ever think fate would lead me down the road I now follow. Someone once told me that God laughs at the plans we mortals make.

Anyone who knows me at all, and who has read this book thus far, cannot doubt the deep love I possess for my wife. I take consolation in the knowledge that I have done all I can for her, and I still continue to do so, but as I learned in the support group, life goes on, and time grows shorter.

What is love, I asked myself? It was a confusing and troubling question, and I agonized over it for quite a while. After much thought and soul searching, an analogy entered my mind that I felt explained it quite well: A couple marries and has a child. This child is everything to them, and they love it with all their hearts. Time goes by, and they have a second child. Consider this, in order to love this child, must they take away some of the love they have for their first child? Of course not. No matter how many children they have, there will always be room for a heart full of love for all of them.

Love is an emotion that you never run out of. It is a bottomless well that never runs dry, and loving someone new does not mean you have to love someone else less. Perhaps I was rationalizing, but I think I understood myself better, and any guilt I may still have been feeling continued to slowly fade away.

I knew I would always love my wife, no matter what, and see to it that she was well taken care of for as long as I, or she, lived. There are many types of love as we all know. Perhaps my love for her had transformed from one of romance, to one of compassion, a love filled with so many wonderful memories of who she once was but who, I am grudgingly forced to admit, no longer exists.

A doorway has appeared in that frightening cement room of my dreams. The doorway enabled me to escape from my loneliness into a pleasant world of music, dancing, and companionship. We all see life differently, and there are many ways to escape from your own personal cement room.

The important thing is to get off the couch and try to make every day count. Arrange to find time for yourself, for you also have a right to enjoy life. It can be done.

There are many agencies that will aid you with respite care and allow you to get involved with many social activities such as your church. For others, a weekly card game, or perhaps bowling, golf, or some other sport. Ladies' clubs, or men's clubs. Get involved.

Go out to dinner with friends when invited and do not worry about being a fifth wheel. Be cheerful, misery loves company, but company does not love misery. Do not ever lose your sense of humor.

Remember the old adage, "Yesterday is gone, today is a gift, and tomorrow may never come."

Keep your face to the sun, and the shadows will fall behind you. There can be a rainbow at the end of the road.

My Sweet Terry Is Gone Now

God saw she was getting tired, and a cure was not to be.
So he put his arms around her and whispered, "Come with me."
With tearful eyes, we watched her suffer and saw her fade away.
Although we loved her dearly, we knew she could not stay.
A golden heart stopped beating hardworking hands to rest.
God broke our hearts to prove to us he only takes the best.
The Alzheimer's she suffered from she suffers from no more.
She is in a better place as she walks through God's pearly door.